Good Food For Kids

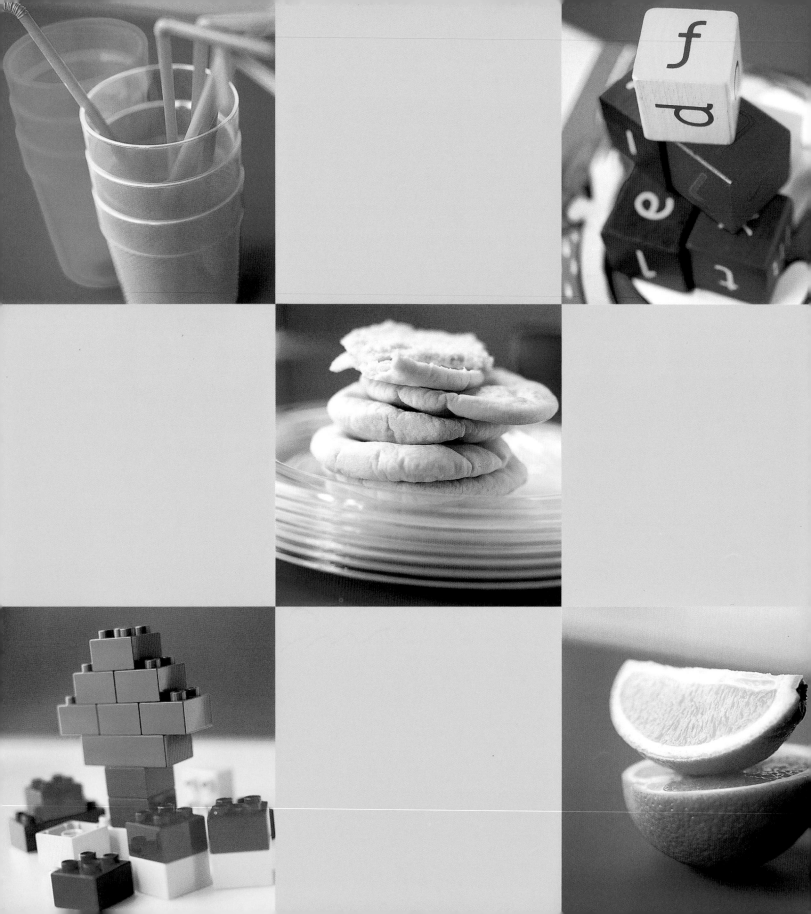

hamlyn

Good Food For Kids

Dr Penny Stanway

First published in Great Britain in 2000 by Hamlyn
a division of Octopus Publishing Group Limited
2-4 Heron Quays
London E14 4JP

First published in paperback in 2003

Photography and design copyright © 2000, 2003 Octopus Publishing Group Limited
Text copyright © 2000 Penny Stanway

ISBN 0600 60882 4

British Library Cataloguing-in-Publication Data
A catalogue record for this book is available from the British Library

Produced by Toppan, Hong Kong
Printed in China

Commissioning Editor: **Nicola Hill**
Creative Director: **Keith Martin**
Executive Art Editor: **Mark Winwood**
Designer: **Louise Griffiths**
Production Controller: **Lisa Moore**
Home Economist: **Dagmar Vesely**
Stylist: **Helen Trent**
Additional Recipes: **Joanna Farrow**
Children's Portrait Photographer: **Peter Pugh-Cook**

NOTES
All recipes serve 4 to 6 depending on the age and appetite of family members, except
where otherwise indicated.

Standard level spoon measures are used in all recipes.
1 tablespoon = one 15 ml spoon
1 teaspoon = one 5 ml spoon

Both metric and imperial measures are given for the recipes. Use one set of measures
only, not a mixture of both.

Ovens should be preheated to the specified temperature. If using a fan assisted oven,
follow the manufacturer's instructions for adjusting the time and temperature. Grills
should also be preheated.

Medium eggs should be used unless otherwise specified.

Use full-fat milk unless otherwise stated.

Pepper should be freshly ground unless otherwise specified.

Fresh herbs should be used unless otherwise stated. If unavailable, use dried herbs as
an alternative but halve the quantities stated.

Ideally stock should be freshly made; recipes for vegetable and chicken stock appear on
pages 51 and 84 respectively. Alternatively buy a carton of fresh stock, ensuring it is salt-
free for under-ones.

Food Pyramid: USDA and DHHS

Contents

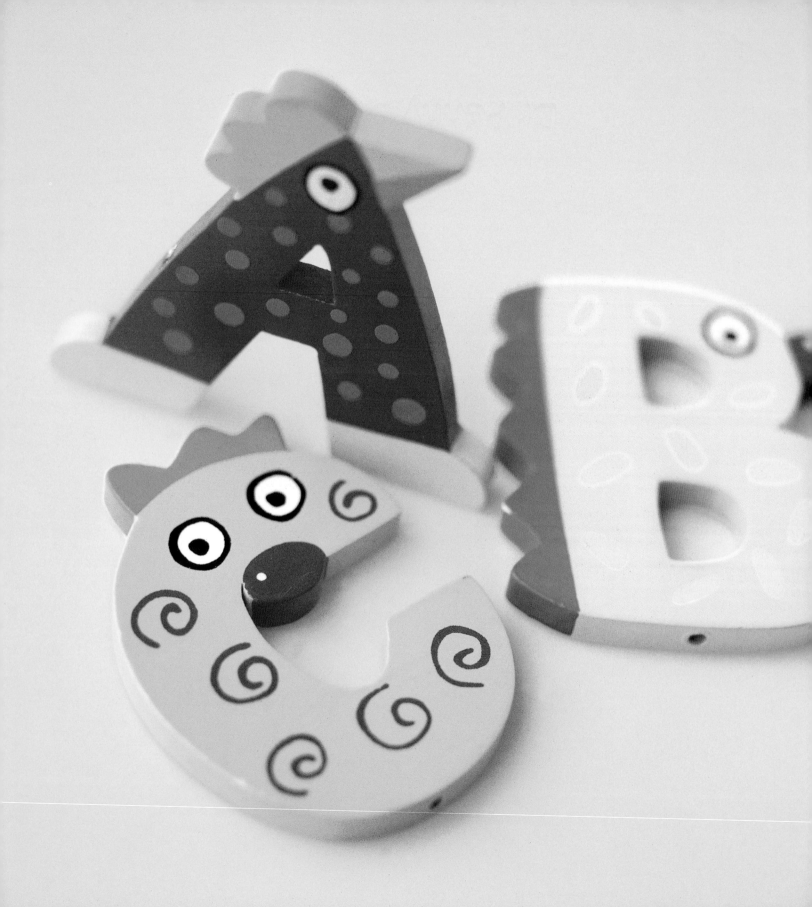

introduction

Good food is one of life's great pleasures for everyone – from the smallest breastfed baby to the most elderly member of the family. It's also vital for good health. We are, after all, what we eat. So, one of our most important roles as parents is to give our children a variety of food they'll enjoy and that will help them grow up healthy, fit and full of energy.

This can prove to be a challenge. Initially, as a first-time mum, you have to learn when and how to introduce 'solids', what to offer, and how to ease the baby's progress towards eating the same food as the rest of the family. Secondly, you may well have a toddler or young child who is fussy about food. Thirdly, we are all subject to media food scare reports and left to question which foods really are good for us. And lastly, as role models to our children, we may need to improve our own eating habits before we can guide our children towards a healthy diet.

What we all want – as I know from bringing up my own three children and helping thousands of mothers over the years to feed theirs – is sound, simple, practical information and encouragement. And that's what you'll find in the first part of this book.

The second part provides a selection of tempting family recipes for every sort of meal, as well as ideas for packed lunches and parties. You will also find suggestions on how to adapt each recipe for babies under one. That way everyone gets to enjoy good, home-cooked food, and life is easier for you.

It's important to realise that feeding your family well will reduce their risk of certain illnesses when they are grown up too. This is partly because healthy eating habits learnt now will probably stay with them in adult life. And having a healthy diet as an adult is proven to reduce the risk of problems such as adult-onset diabetes, several sorts of cancer, gum disease, osteoporosis (which makes the bones fragile), and arterial disease (the main cause of heart attacks and strokes).

Studies are increasingly finding that the way we feed our babies and young children can have effects that last way into adult life. This is one of the most exciting areas of modern nutritional research and emphasises the importance of getting your children off to a good start.

Penny Stanway

WHAT IS A HEALTHY BALANCED DIET?

A well-balanced diet has enough nutrients and calories to meet a child's needs. It lays the foundation of a lifetime of good health, and it helps your child stay healthy and full of energy.

Babies need only milk for the first 4-6 months, and breast milk is undoubtedly best. You can start introducing tastes of solids as early as 4 months if your baby seems ready. However, hungry babies of 4 or 5 months may simply want more milk, so don't rush in with solids too soon. If you want to increase your milk supply, breastfeed more often and, perhaps, for longer, and over the next 2 to 3 days you'll begin making more milk. It's wise to wait no longer than 6 months before offering solids.

Milk is a baby's most important food for the first year. After that, the baby continues to make the transition from a predominantly milk diet to what the rest of the family eats, though milk is still an important source of nourishment. This is partly because it contains quite a lot of fat, and under-fives need proportionately more fat than older children and adults do.

THE FOOD PYRAMID

Providing a nutritious and balanced diet is easy with the help of the food pyramid. All you need to do is:
• Give the different food groups in the proportions shown
• Choose a variety of foods from each layer
• Go by the suggested number and size of helpings

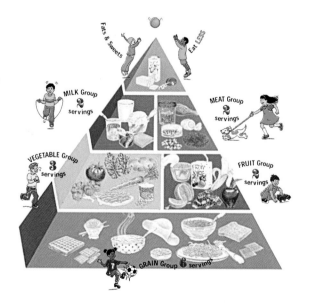

USING THE FOOD PYRAMID

The food groups which make up the 4 layers of the pyramid are: grains; vegetables and fruits; proteins; fats and added sugar. When balancing the family's diet, it helps to think of foods as belonging to one of these 4 main groups.

The pyramid shows the proportion of food from each group to offer your family and eat yourself each day. It won't matter if you don't stick to it exactly – or even if you occasionally go very astray – but it gives you good general guidelines.

Each layer represents a group of foods. The lower the layer, the more foods you need from that group for a healthy diet. So, the foods in the bottom layer – the grains – should form the bulk of your family's food. We should have only a little of the foods at the top of the pyramid – the fatty and sugary things – but many of us consume too much of them.

APPETITE AND PORTION SIZE

Few children want to eat the same amount every day. Our appetite changes according to how active we are, how we feel, how hot or cold it is, and whether others are eating with us. So if your child eats more or less than suggested, don't be alarmed. Look at the eating pattern over the course of a week; if this corresponds roughly to the proportions in the pyramid and your child is growing, feeling and looking well, the number and sizes of helpings don't much matter.

The following guide to the food pyramid layers includes indications of portion size. Note that the cup used for some portion measures has a 250 ml (8 fl oz) capacity.

GRAINS (the first layer)

These include wheat, barley, oats, corn and rice, as well as less popular grains such as rye, millet and sorghum.

A STANDARD CHILD HELPING IS:
• 1 slice of bread
• ½ cup of cooked pasta
• ½ cup of cooked porridge
• 25 g (1 oz) breakfast cereal
• ½ cup of cooked rice

However, children under the age of four generally eat smaller helpings. Be guided by common sense when you're dishing out food – if a child regularly leaves half a standard helping of cereal, for example, give only half as much next time. Remember to offer a variety of grains, not just wheat.

Under-ones may go from eating one small helping a day at first, to having as many as three, or even four, by the end of the first year. This may sound a lot, but babies grow faster during their first year than at any other time, and they use a lot of calories. Some babies prefer to get most of their nourishment from milk until well past their first birthday.

1 year-olds may eat as many as 3-4 small daily helpings. The guidelines aren't strict because a lot of their nourishment still comes from milk.

2-6 year-olds can be offered 6 daily helpings. 2-3 year-olds will probably want small helpings, but 4 year-olds often eat standard-sized helpings. If your child can't eat this many helpings of grains, you can make up the balance by offering starchy choices from other layers of the pyramid, such as potatoes, carrots, peas, beans and bananas.

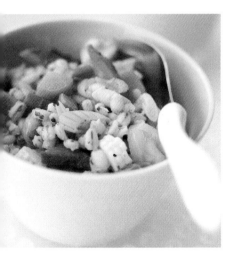

Older children will generally eat 6-11 helpings depending on their appetite.

Six helpings a day may sound a lot but it's easily achieved, for example, you could offer:
• A bowl of breakfast cereal
• A piece of cornbread (see page 133) for a mid-morning snack
• Pasta (such as Tuna & Pasta Gratin, page 49) for lunch
• A slice of toast for tea
• Barley Pot (see page 91) for supper
• Fruit Crumble (see page 104) for dessert

VEGETABLES AND FRUIT (the second layer)

These are rich in nutrients, especially vitamins and minerals; they are also an excellent source of the fibre and antioxidants which help to protect the body against diseases. Offer children a variety of vegetables including starchy ones, like potatoes, carrots and swede; green leafy vegetables, such as cabbage, broccoli and spinach; yellow-orange vegetables, such as carrots, pumpkin, sweet potato and squash.

Give children plenty of different fruits, too, including citrus fruits, like oranges and grapefruit; yellow-orange fruits, such as mangoes and apricots; berry fruits and tree fruits, like apples, pears and plums. Aim to have green leafy vegetables several times a week – most children favour broccoli, but there are plenty

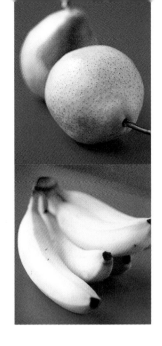

of other options. Beans, peas and lentils are included in the third layer of the pyramid because they are rich in protein, but if your child won't eat enough other vegetables, you can include them in this layer's choices.

A STANDARD CHILD HELPING IS:

• 1 cup of raw leafy vegetable, like lettuce or spinach
• ½ cup of other raw vegetables, or cooked vegetables
• 1 medium apple, pear or orange
• 1 melon wedge or slice of pineapple
• ½ grapefruit, mango or papaya
• ½ cup of fresh grapes or berries
• ½ cup of canned or stewed fruit
• ¼ cup of dried fruit
• 175 ml (6 fl oz) vegetable or fruit juice

Under-fours will probably want smaller helpings, so be guided by common sense.

Under-ones may progress to 3 or 4 small daily helpings by the end of the first year, but don't worry if they don't. The main reason for giving babies fruit and vegetables is to introduce them to the tastes and textures.

One year-olds may have 3 or 4 small daily helpings, but don't be too concerned if they don't. Encourage a child to enjoy fruit and vegetables when they are relaxed and offer them a variety.

Children over two may eat 5 daily helpings; 2-3 year-olds will probably want small helpings.

Five helpings a day may sound a lot but they soon add up, for example, you could offer:
• A glass of orange juice, plus Baby Bear's Big Breakfast (see page 34) to start the day
• A wholemeal cracker thinly buttered and topped with some fine shavings of cheese and halved cherry tomatoes mid-morning
• Frittata (see page 58) with spinach and pepper, for lunch
• A piece of fruit at teatime
• Fish Stir-fry (see page 80) for supper
• Raspberry Fool (see page 97) for dessert

This would bring the total to 6 helpings.

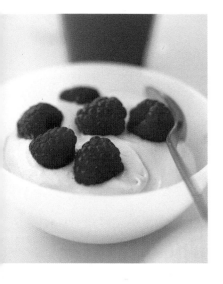

PROTEIN-RICH FOOD (the third layer)

These include dairy foods – milk, cheese, fromage frais and yogurt; other animal protein foods – meat, poultry, game, fish and eggs; and vegetable protein foods – beans and their products, such as tofu, peas and lentils.

A STANDARD CHILD HELPING IS:

- 50-75 g (2-3 oz) of meat, fish or cheese
- 2 medium eggs
- ½ cup cooked beans or lentils

Offer smaller helpings to under-fours, being guided by what your child will eat.

Under-twos may eat 1 or even 2 small daily helpings of meat, poultry, game, fish, eggs or beans. The milk they drink still provides much of their protein requirement.

2-6 year-olds can have 2 helpings of milk or other dairy food, plus 2 helpings of meat, poultry, game, fish, eggs or beans each day. Over-twos can have half-fat (semi-skimmed) cow's milk, but don't give skimmed milk to a child under 5 years of age.

Older children may well want 2-3 daily helpings of dairy food, plus 2-3 helpings of meat, poultry, game, fish, eggs or beans each day.

Teenagers need 3 daily helpings of dairy food.

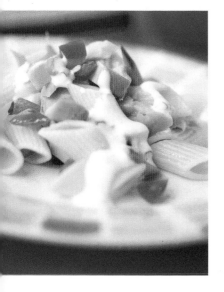

On a weekly basis offer children over 2 years – and adults – 2-3 helpings of beans or peas a week, plus about 3 helpings of oily fish a week. Limit red meat (beef, lamb and pork) to no more than 3 helpings a week, because it contains a relatively high proportion of saturated fat. Although young children need relatively more fat than adults, it's still wise not to overdo saturated fat.

FOODS HIGH IN FATS AND ADDED SUGAR (the fourth layer)

These include vegetable oils, butter, cream cheese, cream, mayonnaise, sugar, cakes, biscuits, sweets, honey, jam, maple syrup, ice cream and soft drinks.

Aim to minimise these fatty and sugary foods when cooking for your family, because they are very concentrated sources of fat and sugar. Children certainly do need fats, but they are present in many other valuable foods, including milk, cheese, yogurt, meat, chicken, oily fish, eggs, nuts and seeds. Neither children nor adults should have much in the way of concentrated sources of fats from the fourth layer.

We don't actually need any added sugar, but it does taste good. If you give your family sugary foods, favour low-sugar products like low-sugar jam, and use less sugar in cooking. Where the recipes in this book contain sugar, the amount is usually less than in other comparable recipes. Sugary foods are all right in moderation, but it's best to give under-ones very little – if, indeed, you give any at all – so they don't learn to crave very sweet foods. Preferably, give sugary foods after a meal so they don't spoil a child's appetite, and make sure your child's teeth are brushed afterwards.

QUALITY AND QUANTITY

Some children get plenty of calories but not enough of certain nutrients. The most likely problems are:
- A lack of calcium, iron and folic acid. Check out the foods that contain these nutrients (see pages 13-14) and ensure your child eats enough of them.
- Too much refined carbohydrate in the form of white bread and pasta, most biscuits, cakes and breakfast cereals, white rice, and added sugar. Choose wholegrain bread, pasta, flour, cereals and rice, and cut down on sugar.
- Not enough vegetables and fruit.
- Too much fat. Under-fives need a relatively large amount, and they generally obtain most of this from milk. However, many older children in particular eat too much fat, especially the 'hidden' fat in biscuits, crisps, fried food, ice cream, puddings, pastry, chocolate and cakes.
- Too much saturated fat. Choose lean meat and trim off visible fat. Use the minimum of oil and fat when cooking. Once your children are over 2 years old, consider buying semi-skimmed (half-fat) rather than full-fat milk, and try introducing other reduced-fat dairy foods.

NUTRIENTS and foods they are found in

You don't need to be a scientist to plan well-balanced, nutritious and delicious meals for your family, but it's useful to have some understanding of the nutritional values of foods. The food pyramid (on page 8) makes planning a balanced diet easier, though at times, you may require more detail. For example, you may want to know which foods can help cure a common ailment (see pages 28-31). If so, use this information to find out what the individual nutrients do, and which foods are the best sources.

PROTEINS

Found mainly in: meat, fish and eggs; breast milk and dairy products; peas, beans and nuts.

What they do: Proteins are made up of amino acids, and are the body's building blocks. Children need proteins for growth, and we all need them for good digestion, energy production, and the formation of new cells to replace those that are worn out or damaged.

Protein-containing foods supply a range of amino acids. Meat, fish, breast milk, dairy foods and eggs contain the whole range of essential amino acids but non-animal protein foods, such as beans and peas, don't. However, a mixture of plant proteins will provide all of the essential amino acids. So, provided your family has a variety of protein-containing foods each day, they will get all they need, even if they're vegetarian (see page 22).

The amino acids, arginine, lysine and tryptophan, feature in the Foods for Common Ailments section (pages 28-31). Arginine is present in meat, fish, dairy food, eggs and beans, and also in nuts, seeds, chocolate and wholegrains. Lysine is found in peas, beans and lentils, and also in cabbage and potatoes. Tryptophan is present in meat, fish, dairy food, eggs and beans, and also cauliflower, potatoes, bananas, dates, nuts, seeds and wholegrains.

CARBOHYDRATES

There are 3 forms of carbohydrate: sugars, such as fruit sugar (fructose), milk sugar (lactose), and the sort of sugar you add to food (sucrose); starches; and fibre. Starches and fibre are called complex carbohydrates.

SUGARS

Found mainly in: fruit, vegetables, honey, breast milk, dairy foods.

What they do: Our body can use sugars as a ready source of energy. The sugar you find in packets or sweetened foods is extracted from sugar cane or sugar beet. I call it 'added sugar' to distinguish it from the intrinsic natural sugar that you get, along with fibre, when you eat fruit and vegetables. Honey and maple syrup are very rich in natural sugar but don't contain any fibre, so their sugars behave more like added sugar in the body.

Giving naturally sweet fruits, vegetables and milk is the best way to include sweetness in your family's diet. However, it's fine to give food that contains added sugar sometimes, as long as the diet remains balanced. Remember, though, that added sugar provides 'empty calories', meaning it's only an energy source, and contains no other nutrients. So don't give your children too much, or you'll spoil their appetite for foods that are more nutritious, and you may encourage them to become overweight. Added sugar is also a major cause of tooth decay, while sugars in fruit and vegetables tend to be washed from the teeth by the increased saliva flow as they are chewed.

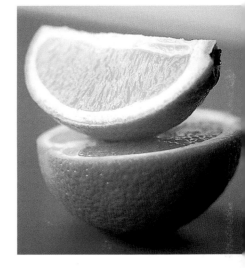

If you give your children foods containing added sugar, it's a good idea always to include meat, fish, eggs, milk, cheese, yogurt, oil, butter, nuts, vegetables, fruits or oats in the same meal. These are 'low-GI' foods (see page 31) which delay the absorption of sugar and so prevent the blood-sugar level rising too quickly, and falling equally fast.

Recipes that include added sugar together with low-GI foods include Flapjacks (see page 128), Pink Tubby Custard (see page 103), and Carrot Cakes (see page 130).

STARCHES

Found mainly in: grains, like wheat, oats, barley, rye, rice, corn (maize), buckwheat, millet, sorghum; beans, peas and lentils; root vegetables, such as carrots, parsnips, potatoes, beetroot, swede, turnips, yams and sweet potatoes; bananas and plantains.

What they do: Starches are broken down into sugars and used for energy.

Recipes rich in starches include Macaroni Mountain (see page 47), Pizzas (see page 52-4) and Barley Pot (see page 91).

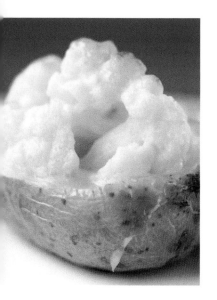

FIBRE (NON-STARCH POLYSACCHARIDE)

Found in: fruit, vegetables, nuts, seeds and wholegrains.

What it does: Fibre encourages a healthy hormone balance, and helps prevent constipation. White flour, white rice, and white pasta have had their fibre removed, and are called refined carbohydrates. Wholemeal or wholegrain flour, bread and breakfast cereal, brown pasta and brown rice still contain their natural fibre. Ideally, you should favour unrefined carbohydrates and serve refined carbohydrates only with other fibre-rich foods, such as fruit and vegetables. Another tip is to use half wholemeal and half white flour in recipes calling for flour, rather than all white flour.

Recipes rich in fibre include Baby Bear's Big Breakfast (see page 34), Baked Potatoes with Cauliflower Cheese (see page 72) and Fruit Kebabs (see page 98).

FATS

These are made of saturated and unsaturated fatty acids (which I shall refer to simply as 'fats'). There's a mixture in most fatty foods, but their proportions vary a great deal and it's important to get a good balance. Many older children in westernised countries grow up eating too much fat, too much saturated fat, and too little of one particular group of unsaturated fats – omega-3 fats. But it's easy to avoid these pitfalls if you know a little bit about fats.

What they do: Fats are a rich source of energy and often of fat-soluble vitamins too, but a high intake may lead to obesity. A good balance of fats in adequate quantities boosts immunity, helps prevent dry skin, rashes and certain cancers, and helps keep muscles, nerves and arteries healthy.

SATURATED FATS

Found in: meat, eggs, milk and other dairy products; margarine and white cooking fat.

Whole-fat (full-fat) milk and other dairy products contain more saturated fat than half-fat or low-fat types. Under-twos need whole-fat milk and dairy products for the other essential nutrients they provide and while 2-5 year-olds can have half-fat products, they shouldn't have low-fat ones. A high intake of saturated fats in later life can increase the risk of a high blood cholesterol level and heart disease, so you should aim to reduce your children's intake as they get older.

POLYUNSATURATED FATS (OMEGA-3 AND OMEGA-6 FATS)

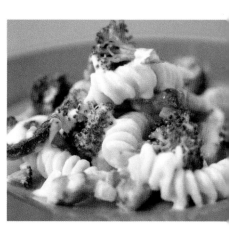

A healthy person can make the whole family of each of these two groups of fats if they eat foods containing the 'parent' fat of each group. So the 'parent' omega-3 and omega-6 fats are called essential fats. However, many children are short of omega-3s.

Essential omega-6 fat is found in: avocados, beans and soya oil; corn and corn oil; seeds and seed oils – including sunflower and rapeseed (canola) oil; and soft margarines.

Essential omega-3 fat is found in: green leafy vegetables (including broccoli); beans; wholegrains; meat from grass-fed animals; chicken; sweet potato; walnuts and their oil; pumpkin seeds and their oil; rapeseed (canola) oil; olives and olive oil. Breast milk is also rich in essential omega-3 fat, which is one reason why it's good to go on breastfeeding beyond 6 months.

Non-essential omega-3 fat is found in: cold-water oily fish, such as herrings, sardines and salmon; these are especially rich sources if fresh or frozen rather than canned. Most of us make these particular omega-3s from foods rich in essential omega-3 fat. However, a poor diet or any other physical or mental stress can interfere with this process, in which case fish is important.

What omega-3 and omega-6 fats do: A good balance discourages allergies, and helps prevent some types of depression by boosting the level of serotonin (a substance that helps messages pass along nerves). It can also help keep arteries and blood healthy, reduce dry skin and psoriasis, and help prevent respiratory infections and certain behaviour problems. It may even ease the symptoms of cystic fibrosis.

Omega-3 rich dishes include Coconut Mackerel with Sweet Potato (see page 82) and Curly Coconut Pasta (see page 39).

MONO-UNSATURATED FATS

Found mainly in: olives and olive oil; avocados; most nuts and their oils; and sesame seeds and their oil.

What they do: These fats help keep the arteries healthy and protect against arterial disease in later life.

MINERALS

You and your family need a variety of minerals to strengthen bones and teeth, release energy, and help control the composition of body fluids and cells.

CALCIUM

Found mainly in: milk, other dairy products and eggs; canned sardines or salmon; shellfish; green leafy and root vegetables; beans, peas and lentils; nuts and seeds; wholegrain foods.

What it does: Calcium works with another mineral, magnesium, to promote the wellbeing of every cell. It helps muscles contract and is essential for strong bones and teeth. If the diet lacks calcium, the body removes some from the bones. When the calcium level of the diet increases, calcium re-enters the bones. Calcium is necessary for healthy hormone action, blood, blood pressure, energy production, nerves, and vitamin B12 absorption.

Recipes rich in calcium include Rice Pudding with Fruit Sauce (see page 106), Baked Plum Custard (see page 102) and Gotta Lotta Bottle (see page 77).

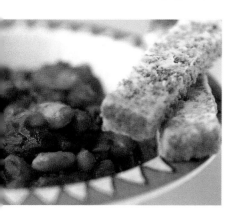

CHROMIUM

Found mainly in: shellfish; liver; dairy products; mushrooms; beans; wholegrain foods.

What it does: Chromium helps keep the blood-sugar level steady.

Recipes which are good sources of chromium include Every Flavour Beans (see page 69) and Veggie Burgers (see page 71).

IODINE

Found mainly in: fish; dairy products and eggs; fruit and vegetables (other than those in the cabbage family); pineapple; raisins; wholegrain foods.

What it does: Iodine enables production of the thyroid hormone.

IRON

Found mainly in: meat, especially liver; shellfish; egg yolk; green leafy vegetables; elderberries; beans and peas; nuts and seeds; prunes and apricots; wholegrain foods.

What it does: Iron is essential for the production of certain enzymes, and haemoglobin (the oxygen-carrying pigment in red blood cells). It's also needed for immunity, energy production, liver function, and the protection of cells when the body is stressed.

Recipes rich in iron include Frittata (see page 58), Magic Mince (see page 90) and Easy Peasy Lasagne (see page 51).

MAGNESIUM

Found mainly in: meat; fish; eggs; green leafy vegetables; mushrooms; beans and peas; nuts and seeds; wholegrain foods; dark chocolate.

What it does: Magnesium works with calcium (see left). It also helps with energy production; the manufacture of insulin, vitamin B and proteins; and the removal of waste products.

Recipes rich in magnesium include Pocket Omelette (see page 35) and Chocolate Puddle Pud (see page 107).

POTASSIUM

Found mainly in: vegetables and fruit, especially avocados, bananas, potatoes, green leafy vegetables, tomatoes and beans; and nuts.

What it does: Potassium helps to regulate the body's acidity level and fluid balance. It is also needed for transporting carbon dioxide; for keeping cell membranes, nerves and muscle tissues healthy; and for the production of proteins.

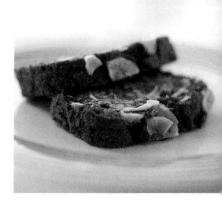

Recipes rich in potassium include Finger Fruits & Yogurt (see page 33), and Banana Teabread (see page 129).

SELENIUM

Found mainly in: meat; fish and shellfish; dairy products and egg yolk; green leafy vegetables, mushrooms and garlic; beans and peas; nuts; wholegrain foods.

What it does: Selenium is an antioxidant, which means it helps prevent damage to cells from substances called free radicals.

These are formed by such things as too much sunbathing, breathing smoke-filled air, eating a poor diet, over-exercising, and feeling stressed. Selenium is also needed to activate thyroid hormones, and in the manufacture of prostaglandins.

Recipes rich in selenium include Fish Stir-fry (see page 80) and Popeye's Pork (see page 64).

ZINC

Found mainly in: red meat, especially liver; fish and shellfish; dairy products and eggs; root and green leafy vegetables; beans and peas; garlic; nuts and seeds; fruit; and wholegrains.

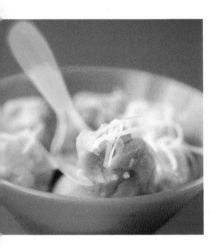

What it does: Zinc is an anti-oxidant that helps to mop up high levels of potentially damaging 'free radicals'. It is vital for growth, energy, the function of prostaglandins and vitamin A, good immunity, and the production of many enzymes, hormones and proteins.

Recipes rich in zinc include Shark Soup (see page 67), Sage & Squash Gnocchi (see page 74) and Carrot Cakes (see page 130).

VITAMINS

These substances are vital for the body to function normally.

VITAMIN A, INCLUDING BETA-CAROTENE

Found mainly in: liver; dairy products and eggs. Many fruits and vegetables are a good source of beta-carotene, especially carrots and other orange, red and yellow ones. Our bodies convert beta-carotene into vitamin A.

What it does: Vitamin A promotes healthy eyesight, growth, immunity and protein manufacture, and helps keep mucous membranes moist. Beta-carotene acts as an antioxidant that helps prevent damage to the cells from free radicals – particles produced by breathing smoke-filled air, eating a poor diet, feeling stressed, and being unwell. It's possible, though unproven, that eating foods rich in vitamin A may help reduce damage to the skin by over-exposure to the sun. Recipes rich in vitamin A include Spinach & Ricotta Puff Pie (see page 93), Traffic Lights (see page 94) and Pumpkin Faces (see page 141).

B VITAMINS

This group of vitamins includes thiamin (B1), riboflavin (B2), niacin (B3), pantothenic acid, pyridoxine (B6), biotin, cyanocobalamin (B12), and folate (folic acid).

Found mainly in: meat, especially liver; fish; dairy products and eggs; beans, peas and lentils; green leafy vegetables; mushrooms; avocados; bananas; nuts and seeds; sprouted seeds; and wholegrains.

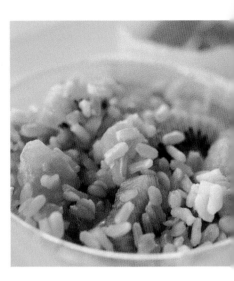

What they do: The vitamins in this group work together to aid growth, metabolism and energy production, and help keep every cell healthy – especially those in blood vessels, muscles and nerves. All of the B vitamins, except B12 and folate, are involved in the release of energy from food. Vitamin B12 is needed for red blood cell formation; calcium, magnesium and selenium metabolism; zinc absorption; and nerve function. Folate (or folic acid) helps keep arteries healthy. It is also vital for the production of the protein in haemoglobin – the pigment in red blood cells. Having enough folic acid before conception and in early pregnancy helps prevent neural tube birth defects. Leafy green vegetables and yeast extract are good sources of folate.

Recipes rich in B vitamins include Fruit & Rice Salad (see page 118) and Banana Teabread (see page 129). Recipes rich in folic acid include Autumn Pasta (see page 45), Curly Coconut Pasta (see page 39) and Coconut Mackerel with Sweet Potato (see page 82).

VITAMIN C

Found mainly in: fruit, especially citrus fruits, blackcurrants and kiwi; and vegetables, especially green leafy ones like broccoli, green peppers and tomatoes.

What it does: This is an antioxidant that helps protect cells from damage by free radicals, particles produced in greater numbers during any physical or mental stress. Vitamin C also helps us absorb iron; aids collagen formation in skin, connective tissues and bone; boosts both immunity and wound healing; and helps us cope with stress.

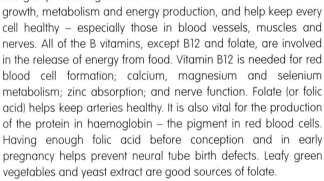

Recipes rich in vitamin C include Finger Fruits & Yogurt (see page 33) and Fresh Fruit Salad (see page 99).

VITAMIN D

Found mainly in: oily fish; dairy products; nuts; cold-pressed vegetable oils. However, our main source of vitamin D is from the effect of sunlight on the skin.
What it does: This helps our body absorb and use calcium, iron and magnesium.

Recipes rich in vitamin D include Pocket Omelette (see page 35), Salmon & Pasta Salad (see page 79) and Toad 'n Roots in the Hole (see page 88).

VITAMIN E

Found mainly in: meat; fish; dairy products and eggs; green leafy vegetables; beans and peas; nuts and seeds and their oils; wholegrains.
What it does: This antioxidant can prolong the life of cells. It also aids fertility and immunity, encourages a healthy balance of prostaglandins (which helps prevent unnecessary inflammation), and helps keep red blood cells healthy.

Recipes rich in vitamin E include Fish Pie (see page 81) and Barbecued Spare Ribs (see page 87).

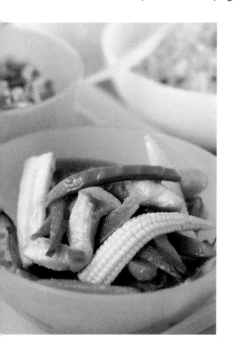

VITAMIN K

Found mainly in: meat, especially liver; egg yolk; green leafy vegetables, broccoli and cauliflower; turnips; tomatoes; bean sprouts and beans; rapeseed (canola) oil and olive oil; and wholegrains. However, our main source of vitamin K is not from food at all but from normal bacteria in the intestine which produce it on a daily basis.
What it does: This vitamin is needed for healthy blood and strong bones.

Recipes rich in vitamin K include Perfect Pizzas and variations (see pages 52-4), and Baby Vegetable & Chicken Stir-fry (see page 57).

OTHER HEALTHY ELEMENTS IN FOOD

PLANT PIGMENTS

Found in: coloured fruits and vegetables; the peel is often the most brightly coloured part and so the richest source.
What they do: Plant pigments counteract inflammation, boost immunity and strengthen tiny blood vessels.

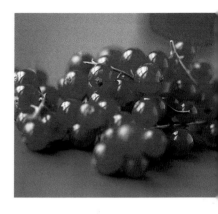

If like many people, you are unfamiliar with plant pigments, you can increase your family's intake simply by giving several different colours of fruits and vegetables each day. Choose from green ones (cabbage, broccoli, lettuce, peas and kiwi fruit), red ones (red cabbage, beetroot, red pepper and raspberries), blue or purple ones (aubergines, blueberries and black grapes), and yellow or orange ones (carrots, swede, squashes and apricots). Buy organic fruit and vegetables, to ensure their skins are free of pesticides, and use unpeeled if possible. Citrus fruit rind is rich in pigments, called citrus flavanoids, but if you intend to use it, it is best to buy organic, unwaxed fruit.

PLANT HORMONES

Found in: beans and bean sprouts; beetroot, cabbage, carrot, celery and fennel; chick peas, lentils and peas; garlic, olives, parsley and sage; potatoes; wholegrain foods; seeds; cherries, plums and rhubarb; and in smaller amounts in other vegetables and fruits.
What they do: Some are sufficiently similar to certain of our own hormones (such as oestrogen) to be able to lock on to hormone receptors on cells, and mimic the action of those hormones. When this happens, it may help to correct a hormone imbalance. Plant hormones aren't very 'strong' compared with our own, so are unlikely to cause problems.

SALICYLATES

Found in: many fruits (especially the peel) and vegetables; seeds; nuts.
What they do: Chemically, these resemble aspirin and can help counteract various sorts of inflammation. So if your child has a feverish infection, for example, give more salicylate-rich foods.

FIRST FOODS

The best food for a young baby is milk, and the best milk is breast milk. Indeed, milk is the most important part of a baby's diet – even after starting solids – for the whole of the first year, and often longer. But you should start offering foods other than milk when your baby is 4 to 6 months old, unless there are allergies in the family, when it's better to wait until 6 months. These other foods are called 'solids', however runny they are.

Give your baby some breast milk or formula first, then offer the food on a spoon, preferably one with a fairly flat bowl. Finish by giving another drink of milk.

Put the laden spoon into your baby's mouth, then gently withdraw it against the upper gum and lip so some of the food stays in the mouth. Your baby may try to suck in some of the food from the spoon. Some inquisitive 6 month-olds like to investigate by grasping food from their mother's hand or plate. This is fine as long as it's suitable and not too hot.

Many babies love the new sensations of smelling, tasting and swallowing solids – they smack their lips and start looking for more at once – but the experience takes others by surprise. A screwed-up face doesn't mean your baby doesn't like the food, just that it's unfamiliar. So simply wait for a moment, so the baby doesn't feel pressured, then have another go. A lot of the food that goes in the baby's mouth will probably come out again, but you can scoop this up gently from the chin with the spoon.

Never add puréed food to a bottle. Doing this would reduce the amount of liquid the baby drinks from that bottle, which could lead to dehydration.

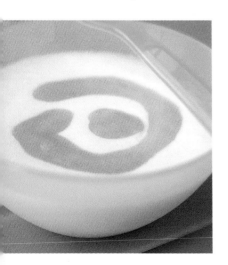

HOMEMADE OR READY-MADE?

Many mothers like to give their babies homemade food most of the time – especially when they can easily adapt what the rest of the family are eating. Jars or tins of commercially prepared food are convenient; for example, when you are on a day out, or on holiday. It's obviously much cheaper to make your own – and if you adapt family recipes, this means your baby quickly gets used to normal family food.

CONSISTENCY

Under 6 months First foods for spoonfeeding must be fairly runny, and soft and smooth enough for your baby to swallow easily. So, you'll need to make purées. Over the first few weeks you can gradually make purées thicker and less smooth.

Over 6 months If you're starting solids now, give relatively runny, soft smooth purées, as above, but

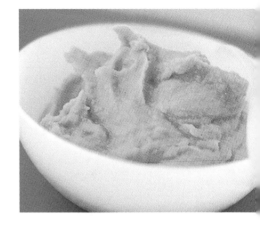

progress quite quickly over the next 2 or 3 weeks to thick, lumpy ones. If your baby has been on purées for some time, start lumpy ones now. Babies of this age soon learn to grind soft lumps of food with their gums. During the next 3 or 4 months, they learn to grind harder lumps with their gums, and as the back teeth emerge, they use these too. However, a lot depends on the type of food and the size of the pieces you give. Meat is difficult to chew, so it needs either to be chopped and blended, or minced, until your baby is around 10 months. After that it may be all right simply cut into very small pieces.

To purée a food you can:
• Mash it
• Push it through a sieve or a mouli
• Whizz it in an electric blender

What you do will depend on the food and your equipment. The only way of making meat smooth is by blending, but you must chop it finely first or it will be stringy.

To thin a savoury purée, add a little of one of the following:
• Expressed breast milk, or formula; this makes a new food more tempting because it adds a familiar flavour and a little sweetness
• Water in which you've cooked vegetables
• Water
• Homemade vegetable stock (see page 51) or chicken stock (see page 84), conveniently frozen in an ice-cube tray so you can use a cube at a time.

To thin a 'sweet' purée, add a little of one of the following:
• Expressed breast milk, or formula; milk makes a new food more attractive because its flavour is familiar
• Water in which you've cooked fruit
• Water

How much to give

The first time you offer solids, give just a little taste from a teaspoon – or even from your (washed) finger. Then if your baby likes it, give a little more. Do the same for each new food. Be sensitive to your baby's appetite and let them guide you as to how much to give.

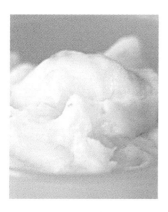

WHICH FOODS TO GIVE
From 4 months

Vegetables:
Avocado
Broccoli
Carrots and other root veg
Cauliflower
Courgette
Squash

Non-gluten grains:
Rice
Corn (such as polenta)
Millet

Other starchy carbohydrates:
Tapioca
Sago

Fruit:
Apple
Apricots
Banana
Pears

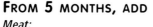

From 5 months, add

Meat:
Chicken
Turkey

From 6 months, add

Dairy foods (full-fat):
Cow's milk
Cheese
Yogurt
Eggs (well cooked)

Grains which contain gluten:
Wheat, barley, rye and oats – as bread and rusks, breakfast

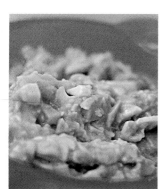

cereals and flour-based sauces

Pulses and legumes:
Peas (tiny tastes can be given earlier)
Lentils, beans and tofu (If beans and lentils make your baby windy, give them for lunch rather than supper, so it doesn't affect your baby's night sleep.)

Other meats and fish:
Lamb
Beef
Pork
Filleted fish

Nuts and seeds:
Ground nuts or seeds (Don't give whole or chopped nuts, or whole seeds, to a child under five, as there is a risk of inhalation or choking.) Note that while true food allergy is rare, it can be serious, and nuts – especially peanuts – are a common trigger.

TIPS FOR THE FIRST YEAR

• *Space out new first foods:* When giving your baby anything other than root vegetables for the first time, don't give it again for 4 days. This lets you see whether your baby develops any symptoms – such as diarrhoea, a runny nose, or a rash – that could suggest an allergy or other sensitivity to that food. It also gives your baby the chance to get used to each new taste.

• *Combining foods:* After the first 2 or 3 weeks, you can give two or more foods in the same meal. However, some babies, just like some adults, prefer foods kept separate, rather than mixed.

• *Avoid added sugar:* The sugar you add to food – rather than the type naturally present in fruits, vegetables and milk – provides 'empty' calories. This means it supplies energy but no other nutrients. Added sugar is best avoided completely for babies of up to 9 months. After that, the very occasional (perhaps weekly) helping of food containing added sugar won't hurt. You may, however, prefer to avoid it for as long as possible – until your baby is old enough to realise that he or she is missing out on something. Remember to clean teeth and gums after any food containing added sugar.

• *Avoid honey:* There is a tiny risk of food poisoning from a toxin which is very rarely present in unpasteurized honey.

• *Avoid salty foods* (see page 25).

• *Avoid added bran:* Don't give your baby breakfast cereals containing added or concentrated bran, as this could prevent iron, calcium and zinc being properly absorbed. Bran is also very filling, which could spoil your baby's appetite.

HOMEMADE FIRST FOODS

The following ideas should provide you with plenty of scope for preparing your baby's own first food. This needn't be a time-consuming chore. Prepare more food than your baby needs and freeze the surplus in convenient small portions. An ice-cube tray is ideal for this. Take out one or more frozen cubes as needed, put in a bowl, cover and allow to defrost at room temperature for an hour or so, or overnight in the refrigerator. If you find you have forgotten to defrost the food in advance, use the microwave. Always reheat defrosted food thoroughly in a saucepan, or in the microwave, then cool to the correct temperature for your baby.

VEGETABLES

For the following, do not add salt to cooking water, or to the purée. If stock is used, it should be homemade and salt-free.

Potato purée: Boil, steam or bake a peeled potato. Drain if appropriate, then mash the potato. Mix in some cooking water, milk or stock. It's easy to produce a smooth purée of potato simply by mashing with a fork. Vary the flavour by using different potatoes and liquids.

Carrot purée: Boil or steam a peeled carrot. Either blend it with a little cooking water, milk or stock, or put it through a mouli or a sieve before adding liquid. (Mashing doesn't produce such a smooth purée.) This sweet, bright orange purée is often popular.

Parsnip purée: Make as for Carrot purée, using parsnip instead of carrot. This gives a sweetish, quite strongly flavoured purée.

Sweet potato purée: Make as for Carrot purée, using sweet potato instead of carrot. The sweet potato can be baked in its skin if preferred, then the flesh scooped out of the skin. This is another sweet, orange purée.

Beetroot purée: Make as for Carrot purée, cooking the beetroot until soft; this takes from 30–60 minutes, depending on its age. This is a dramatically pink purée, and one that's naturally sweet. Don't be alarmed if colour from the beetroot passes through into the urine and stains your baby's nappy pink.

Courgette purée: Simply steam the (unpeeled) courgette for 5-10 minutes until soft, then pass through a sieve, adding a little cooking water, milk or vegetable stock, as required.

Butternut squash purée: Make as for Carrot purée, using butternut squash instead of carrot. To cook the squash, either peel and cut into chunks, then boil or steam; or bake wedges, then scoop the flesh from the skin. This purée is an attractive colour that appeals to babies.

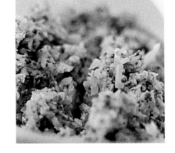

Broccoli or cauliflower purée: Steam broccoli or cauliflower florets for 7-8 minutes or until soft, then purée, adding a little cooking water, milk or stock, as required. Both purées are good first foods but can make a baby windy. If they do, give for lunch rather than supper, so night sleep isn't affected.

FRUIT

Apple purée: Peel, quarter, core and slice 1 eating apple. Cook gently in a little water until soft. Blend to a purée; moisten with a little water or milk. Eating apples are ideal as they are naturally sweet. (Cooking apples would be too tart without added sugar.)

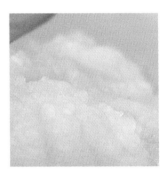

Pear purée: Choose a really ripe, soft pear, and simply peel, core and mash the flesh with a fork, adding a little water or milk if necessary. Or, peel, core and cook a slightly firmer pear in water until soft, then purée with a little water or milk if needed.

Banana purée: Peel the banana, then mash with a fork, adding a little water or milk if needed. This is naturally sweet and popular.

Apricot purée: Choose ripe apricots. Peel, halve and stone very soft apricots, then mash with a fork. Or cook apricots with a little water; halve, stone and blend; then sieve to remove skins.

GRAINS

First rice pudding: Prepare some unsweetened ground ('baby') rice or rice flakes, according to the pack instructions, using water not milk. Then add a teaspoon or so of breast milk or formula. Rice flakes give a slightly less smooth texture than ground rice.

Polenta: This ground cornmeal doesn't contain gluten, so your baby can have it from 4 months. Make the polenta with water or salt-free stock (see page 51), according to the packet instructions. Add a little milk at the end to make it taste more familiar.

Tapioca and sago: These are alternatives to rice pudding. Prepare by cooking in water, according to the packet instructions. Add a little expressed breast milk or formula at the end.

Couscous: As this contains wheat gluten, it is suitable only for babies over 6 months. Make the couscous with water or home-made stock (see page 51), according to the packet instructions. Add a little milk at the end to make it taste more familiar.

Semolina pudding: This is suitable only for babies of 6 months and over, because semolina contains wheat gluten. Prepare the semolina with milk, according to the packet instructions.

OTHER FOODS

Avocado purée: Peel half a ripe avocado, then mash a little of its flesh with a fork, adding a little water, milk or stock. Use at once, as avocado flesh quickly turns brown on contact with air.

Chicken or turkey purée: Offer from 5 months. Blend a little chopped cooked chicken or turkey with some of the cooking juice (if casseroled or poached), vegetable water, stock, water or milk.

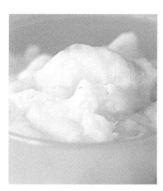

COMBINING FLAVOURS

Once a baby is used to single flavours, try mixtures, such as:
• Carrot and cauliflower
• Courgette and parsnip
• Leek and potato
• Rice and broccoli
• Squash and beetroot
• Sago and apricot
• Pear and semolina

REDUCING THE RISK OF ALLERGY

Your baby has a higher risk of developing an allergy if you, your partner, or a close relative has eczema, allergic asthma, allergic rhinitis (eg hay fever), urticaria, or food allergy. If you are concerned that your baby's risk is high, to reduce it you can:
• Breastfeed exclusively for 6 months, and continue to breastfeed for at least the rest of the first year.
• While breastfeeding, avoid eating dairy foods, eggs, fish and nuts. Seek advice from your doctor or a dietician if necessary, on replacing these foods so your diet remains sound.
• Delay giving your baby the following:
Cow's milk (and 'unhydrolysed soy' formula) until 9 months old
Wheat until 10 months old
Eggs until 11 months old
Cheese, yogurt, oranges, fish and nuts until 12 months old
Peanuts and foods containing peanut oil until 3 years of age
One study found that excluding these foods reduced a baby's risk of allergy from 40% to 14%. However, you should discuss this eating plan with your doctor before implementing it, and carry it out only under the guidance of a doctor or dietician.

When you give one of these foods for the first time, avoid other new foods for the next 4 days, and watch for any unexpected symptoms. A rash, diarrhoea, a runny nose, or more wind or crying than usual might suggest a food allergy or other sensitivity to that food. Discuss the next step with your baby's doctor or other professional health adviser.

'FINGER FOODS'

Try giving an older baby 'finger foods' – foods to hold with the fingers and suck on or chew. Many 6 month-old babies like to try holding food, and by the time they are 8 or 9 months they can often cope very well. Experiment with a large wedge of peeled raw fruit, such as an eating apple. Rusks are another popular finger food; you can make these by baking halved thick slices of wholemeal bread in the oven until hard. Finger foods need to be hard so bits don't break off and make the baby choke. Babies generally eat them by sucking on them until they go mushy.

FIRST DRINKS OTHER THAN MILK

Breast milk or formula is such an important source of nourishment even for a baby who has started solids that you shouldn't give more than a little of any other drink. However, you can give a small drink of water, or of fruit or vegetable juice either as it is, or diluted with water.

MEAL PLANNING

Use the Food Pyramid (see pages 8-10) as a guide to planning your family's meals. To create a well-balanced main meal you may find it helpful to imagine the food on the plate. The largest amount should be a starchy carbohydrate, such as rice, pasta, pizza, couscous, polenta or barley, or the alternatives to these 'grain foods' – potatoes, sweet potatoes, beans, peas or lentils. And the smallest volume should be the protein food – meat, poultry, fish, eggs, beans or peas. Concentrated fats, such as butter and oil, and sugar should be minimal.

The number of daily helpings from each food group I suggest for children of different ages are guidelines rather than set rules. Like all mothers, I know appetites can vary a lot from day to day, so don't worry if your child doesn't always eat the suggested number, or sometimes wants only very small helpings. It's the overall balance over the week that's more important.

MEAL PLANNING FOR UNDER-ONES
1-4 MONTHS

Young babies should obtain all their nourishment from breast milk (or formula).

4 MONTHS

Most babies of this age don't need solids, but it's safe to give them if you think the time is right. However, if there is a family history of allergy (see page 19) it's better to wait until 6 months. Remember that a baby of this age who's hungry probably needs more milk, rather than solids. If you're breastfeeding, boost your milk supply to meet your baby's needs simply by feeding more often, and for longer at each feed. Do this for 2 or 3 days and you should have plenty again. If your baby is extra hungry it may indicate he or she is going through a 'growth spurt'.

To introduce solids, continue with milk feeds as before but choose a time of day, such as lunchtime, to offer a spoonful or so of one of the first foods (suggested on page 17). Two weeks later, offer solids at another time of day, such as breakfast.

5 MONTHS

Milk is still enough for many babies, but you may feel now is the right time to start solids. If you've already started, become more adventurous by combining flavours, making purées thicker and coarser, and, perhaps, adding meat in the form of chicken or turkey. By 5½ months, your baby could be having three different sorts of solids, at breakfast, lunch and supper.

6-12 MONTHS

If you haven't already offered your baby solids, 6 months is the time to do so. Solids become progressively more important during the second half of the first year for most babies. Milk should still provide most of their nourishment. When the nourishment your baby gets from solids begins to equal that from milk, it's important to give a good balance of the different food groups, but this doesn't usually happen until about a year at the earliest. You can offer solids for breakfast, lunch and supper, and, perhaps for a little snack mid-morning and at teatime. Babies vary hugely in how much, and how often they want solids.

Stick with breast milk or formula for drinks, though a small drink of fruit or vegetable juice – diluted if preferred – is fine each day. The only exception is if you're in the process of boosting your breast-milk supply, when all drinks should come from you. Avoid goat's milk, sheep's milk, nut milk or soya milk, as these don't contain the right proportions of nutrients. You can now use full-fat pasteurised cow's milk in the food you make for your baby.

A 6 month-old baby can have some solids for breakfast, lunch and tea. The balance of foods doesn't much matter at this stage, but each day, try offering:
- 2-3 helpings of starchy carbohydrate foods
- 2 helpings of fruit and vegetables (including potatoes, beans or peas if not counted as a starchy alternative to grains)
- 1 helping of a protein-rich food

A 9-12 month baby can be offered the following each day:
- 3-4 helpings of starchy carbohydrate foods
- 3-4 helpings of fruit and vegetables (including potatoes, beans or peas if not counted as a starchy alternative to grains)
- 1-2 helpings of a protein-rich food

If you and the rest of the family eat a healthy, balanced diet and you give your baby some of what you all eat, you won't go far wrong. However, you may need to adjust your recipes

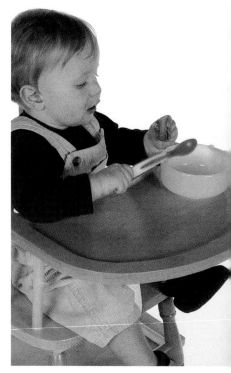

slightly. For example, you must cut out added salt. It's also wise to steer clear of foods containing added sugar (though a little won't hurt occasionally). And it's sensible to use only a hint of any spice at first so a baby can get used to it gradually.

MEAL PLANNING FOR 1-3 YEAR-OLDS

When your baby is 1 year old, milk will probably still be providing at least half of the calories and nourishment needed each day, and perhaps much more, because not all 1 year-olds are eager to eat much in the way of solids. From now on, the solids you give at breakfast, lunch and tea can gradually begin to take over from milk as the main source of nourishment, though milk will continues to be an important food for several years in most young children. If you are breastfeeding, you can give some full-fat cow's milk as well if you like. If you are bottle-feeding, you can give your baby full-fat cow's milk instead of formula now. Cow's milk is fairly low in iron, so if your child is bottle-fed and slow to take to solids, favour iron-rich foods (see page 13) and ask the doctor whether an iron supplement would be a good idea. Breast milk is richer in iron, so iron-deficiency anaemia is unlikely to occur in breastfed 1 year-olds who don't yet eat many solids.

Be relaxed about your child's food intake, because he or she will readily pick up any anxiety on your part. As your baby grows into a toddler, try to offer the same balanced diet as the rest of the family eats. Toddlers shouldn't live on 'nursery food' – bland, smooth, 'white' foods – though like kids of all ages, they may enjoy them from time to time. Young children usually eat better if they are in company, where the attention isn't focused solely on what and how much they eat. So aim for you and your toddler – or the whole family – to eat together whenever possible, and use the time for listening to and learning about each other.

Plan the day's food according to the 'food pyramid' (see pages 8-10), making sure you give your child enough foods containing calcium, iron and vitamins (see pages 13-15), and avoid too many foods that contain added salt and sugar.

Each day, aim to offer:
- 3-4 helpings of starchy carbohydrate foods
- 3-4 helpings of fruit and vegetables (including potatoes, beans or peas if not counted as a starchy alternative to grains)
- 1 helping of a non-dairy protein-rich food
- 2-3 helpings of full-fat milk or other dairy produce (or half-fat for over-twos). Depending on how much other fat your child consumes, you may wish to introduce semi-skimmed milk when they reach the age of two.

MEAL PLANNING FOR OVER 3 YEAR-OLDS

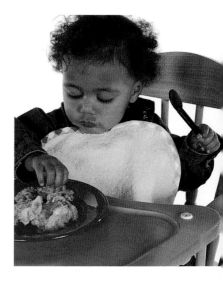

Trust your child to eat what he or she needs. There's every reason to suppose this will happen, provided you don't offer too much food laden with sugar and fat. Never force a child to eat, but don't compensate half an hour afterwards by offering a 'junk-food' snack, high in calories, sugar and/or fat, but with relatively few other nutrients, or the lesson will be that refusing a meal means he or she can then have 'junk food'. Give a healthy snack (see page 22) instead. There's nothing wrong with junk food occasionally, but too much on a regular basis can lead to bad moods and behaviour problems, overweight and nutritional deficiencies.

Each day, aim to offer:
- 6-11 helpings of foods starchy carbohydrate foods – this sounds a lot, but 6 helpings soon adds up (see page 9)
- 5 helpings of fruit and vegetables (including potatoes, beans or peas if not counted as a starchy alternative to grains)
- 2-3 helpings of protein-rich foods

Also, each week, include:
- 2-3 helpings of beans, bean products, or peas (counted either as starchy alternatives to grains, or as vegetables)
- 2-3 helpings of oily fish (counted as protein)
- No more than 3 helpings of beef, lamb or pork, as these red meats contain a relatively high proportion of saturated fats

SCHOOL CHILDREN

A good breakfast helps a child to stay full of energy, and learn well. Choosing what to give your child to take to school for a mid-morning snack can be a challenge because children often want what others are eating. So if this happens to be 'junk' food, they'll probably want a chocolate bar, rather than something more nutritious and better for their teeth (see ideas on page 22). For a young child, try making your healthy 'break' look attractive – perhaps by wrapping it up in shiny cellophane. And chat to other parents to see if you can work together towards sending all the children to school with a nutritious, tooth-friendly snack.

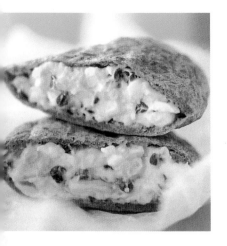

Some children take to school and school lunches like ducks to water. Others need time to adapt to the new environment with its smells, tastes and company. Help your child to adjust by making time to listen, especially straight after school.

If your child takes a packed lunch, turn to pages 108-121 for ideas. Having an attractive, tasty meal will encourage your child to enjoy lunchtime.

Many schoolchildren are very active and need the sort of food and drink that will help keep them full of energy. So for breakfast, break and lunch, include some 'low-GI foods' – that supply a steady source of energy (see page 31).

VEGETARIAN AND VEGAN CHILDREN

If your child is vegetarian, offer plenty of foods containing iron (see page 13) and vitamin B12 (see page 14), as these are the nutrients most likely to be lacking. Also, offer any two of the following three food groups each day:

• Milk – as in fresh milk, cheese or yogurt
• Bread – as in bread, cereals, other grain foods; or actual grains
• Beans – as in beans, peas or lentils

This book includes plenty of vegetarian recipes, including Frittata (see page 58), Veggie Burgers (see page 71), Spinach & Ricotta Puff Pie (see page 93) and Traffic Lights (see page 94).

If your child is a vegan and eats no foods of animal origin at all, check with your doctor that their diet is nutritionally adequate and discuss whether there is a need for any supplement – for example, of vitamin B12. Zen macrobiotic and fruitarian diets are unsuitable for young children.

MAIN MEALS

Breakfast, lunch and supper are the main meals of the day, though many over-ones prefer to eat five or more smaller meals each day. This is easy if you give a snack mid-morning and at teatime, and perhaps a bedtime snack too. All my children were grazers, and it was no problem. One advantage of 'grazing' is that a child doesn't get irritable through hunger between meals. 'Grazing' also works for a child who is 'put-off' by large meals.

BREAKFAST

Some people regard breakfast as the least important meal of the day, but most nutritionists agree it's vital for starting the day right, because breakfast provides fuel and nutrients for the whole body, including the brain. A well-balanced, filling breakfast keeps a child going and, perhaps with a small top-up from a mid-morning snack, prevents a late-morning energy slump. Even a simple poached egg on toast followed by a piece of fruit, for example, will sustain your child. If the choice is a bowl of cereal, encourage them to eat some fruit and protein-rich yogurt, too. Avoid sugar-coated cereals as these are laden with added sugar. Certain special 'energy foods' or 'low-GI foods' (see Tiredness, page 31) will help keep your child well stoked up for a morning's play and learning.

LUNCH

This should be well balanced, and quite substantial, as it may have to provide nutrients and energy to last for some hours. Many school-age children have a long gap between lunch and supper – and some pre-schoolers who attend an afternoon nursery class do too – so include some special 'energy foods' or 'low-GI foods' (see Tiredness, page 31).

SUPPER

This meal can be smaller than the other main meals. Some children sleep better after a supper that's rich in carbohydrate, but not so rich in protein. Any sort of pasta dish (see pages 38-51) is an excellent choice.

SNACKS

Try to make these 'mini meals' nutritious. Avoid cakes and biscuits containing white flour and sugar, or fatty, salt-laden crisps. Instead, offer fresh or dried fruit, or perhaps vegetable sticks with a dip (see page 116). Alternatively give your child a small sandwich (see pages 112-3 for ideas); or a slice of Corn-bread (see page 133); or if you have time, whizz up a fruity milk shake, such as Gotta Lotta Bottle (see page 77).

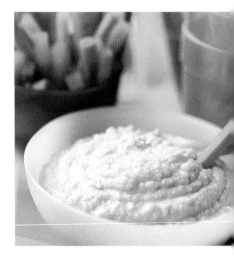

SHOPPING FOR A HEALTHY DIET

Here are some pointers to help you choose what to buy when you are doing your food shopping.

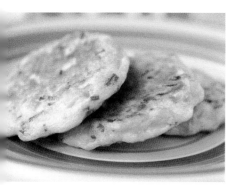

BREAD, PASTA, CEREALS AND OTHER 'GRAIN FOODS'

Foods made from grains or grain flours are generally beneficial, but overall, wholegrains and wholegrain products – including wholemeal flour – are more nutritious. So favour tasty wholemeal bread over white or brown. Consider buying brown rice, which has a delicious nutty taste, too. Wholewheat pasta is another alternative, though you may find as I do, that your family prefers ordinary pasta. Try to use some wholemeal flour in cooking; a mixture of half wholemeal flour and half white works well in most recipes. Some wholegrains, such as pot barley, aren't widely available from supermarkets but you can buy them from healthfood shops.

Ideally, pick out wholegrain breakfast cereals that don't have sugar added, such as muesli or porridge oats, rather than refined and sweetened cereals – which applies to most of the rest. Sugar-coated breakfast cereals are least kind to the teeth.

Corn contains less fibre than other wholegrains, but is particularly versatile – polenta is suitable for young babies, for example; and Sweetcorn Griddle Cakes (page 76) and Cornbread (page 133) are delicious. Other grain foods include semolina and couscous (see page 89); pudding rice and ground rice ('baby' rice). Tapioca, made from the root vegetable cassava, and sago, from the pith of the sago palm, are useful starches, though they are not actually grains.

VEGETABLES AND FRUIT

Fresh fruit and vegetables are the best choice, then frozen and lastly canned. The nutritional difference between fresh and frozen produce is generally small, because food is usually frozen soon after it is harvested. However, canning can destroy up to half of the folic acid in a vegetable. Avoid fruit canned with added sugar, and vegetables canned with added sugar and salt. Don't give any salted canned vegetables to under-ones.

ORGANIC FOODS

Non-organic growers use pesticides several times during the growing season; samples are checked to ensure pesticide residues are within official limits, but some residues remain. The problem is more evident with certain vegetables and fruits, notably carrots, apples and salad leaves. Organic foods are free from pesticides, additives and artificial growth hormones, so you may well prefer to buy these. Organic produce is now readily available in most supermarkets and farmers' markets. It tends to be more expensive, but prices should fall as demand increases.

MILK, YOGURT AND CHEESE

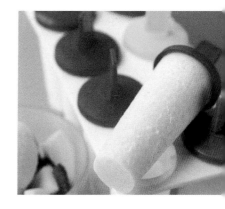

Buying half-fat milk and yogurt, or lower-fat cheeses, is an easy way of lowering the total fat – and specifically the saturated fat – in your family's diet. However, half-fat milk is recommended only for over-twos (and skimmed milk only for over-fives). This is because young children need more fat and fat-soluble nutrients than over-fives for healthy growth and development, and dairy products are a main source of fat in most young children's diets. Provided your family's overall diet isn't too fatty, you may prefer to let everyone continue to eat whole-fat cheese and yogurt, perhaps switching to semi-skimmed milk – it's all a question of balance. Avoid UHT (ultra-heat-treated) yogurts as these contain no gut-friendly bacteria.

FATS AND OILS

Use concentrated fats and oils only in moderation. Butter tastes good and comes in 'spreadable' types. However, it's high in saturated fat, as are hard margarines and white cooking fats. Soft margarines are lower in saturated fat but contain 'trans fats' that behave like saturated fat. Olive oil spreads, however, are free from 'trans fats'. For cooking, I recommend the following oils:
• Extra-virgin olive, rapeseed (canola), walnut or pumpkin seed oil – rich in omega-3s (see page 12)
• Corn, sunflower or rapeseed (canola) oil (again) – rich in omega 6s (see page 12)
Favour omega-3-rich oils for salad dressings and for most cooking purposes.

COOK-CHILLED MEALS, AND OTHER 'PROCESSED FOODS'

Home-cooked meals usually taste better than ready-prepared ones. Many 'shop meals' and 'processed' foods such as mayonnaise or biscuits are high in fat, so read the labels carefully. Many are called 'low fat', when they should be called 'lower fat'. For example, removing fat so a product has 40 g per 100 g instead of 60 g doesn't make it 'low fat'. It may be 'lower fat', but it is still very fatty. No food with a fat content over 4 g per 100 g is really a low-fat one.

DRINKS

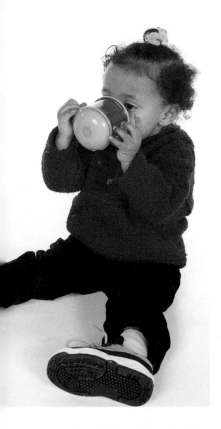

Most children like fruit juice, and some like vegetable juices. Juice is a good way of providing one daily helping of fruit or vegetables. Fresh juice is more nutritious and delicious than reconstituted, and that which is freshly squeezed at home is best of all. If you give your child more than one helping of fruit juice a day, dilute it half and half with water. It's better for a child to get most of their fruit and vegetables intact – with their fibre – than in the form of juice.

Squashes, crushes, fizzy drinks and still soft drinks contain – among other things – added sugar or an artificial sweetener such as aspartame or saccharine. These aren't ideal everyday drinks for young children, so give them only occasionally, if at all.

Cow's milk is fine, but not vital – except for those over-ones who are no longer breastfed or formula-fed, and aren't eating enough solids to nourish them completely. If your over-two doesn't like milk, try water or fruit juice, but as cow's milk is a good source of protein, fat and calcium, discuss with your doctor which other foods your child needs to replace these nutrients.

SNACKS

Supermarkets display shelf after shelf of snacks such as potato crisps, corn puffs and nachos. Salted varieties are totally unsuitable for under-ones. Also, because these snacks are high in fat, they should be given to over-ones only as part of a balanced diet – and then not more than once a day. Instead, consider healthier options (see page 22). Neither whole or chopped nuts, nor whole seeds, are suitable for under-fives because of the risk of inhalation. Smooth peanut butter is fine as a spread, as long as peanut allergy isn't a possibility. However, some schools forbid peanut butter or peanuts in school, to protect any peanut-allergic child who might touch or share them.

FOOD HYGIENE AND STORAGE

Always give your baby or young child only food that looks and smells good. Throw it away if it's at all doubtful – at best it won't taste nice. At worst it could cause gastroenteritis or food poisoning – conditions that can be serious in a young child. The most risky foods from this point of view are meat (raw or cooked), paté, fish, dairy products, cook-chilled ready meals, and frozen food that has been allowed to thaw, then refrozen.

Here are some tips to help keep food in good condition:
• Refrigerate or freeze meat, poultry, fish and dairy products
• Defrost frozen meat, poultry and fish in the refrigerator
• Keep raw meat, poultry and fish separate from other foods, and never allow their juices to drip on to other food
• Keep dried foods in sealed containers, and frozen food in airtight containers
• Cook meat and poultry thoroughly, until the juices run clear when you test the meatiest part with a knife
• Refrigerate leftovers at once and only for 1-2 days, or throw them away
• Never give your family food past its 'use-by' date.
• Don't let the fridge temperature rise above 4°C (40°F), or the freezer temperature above -18°C (0°F)
• Don't leave foods in the freezer too long. Use them in rotation, and check your freezer manual to see how long each food can safely be frozen
• Don't use the same chopping board for cutting raw meat other foods. After preparing raw meat and fish, wash your hands, knife and chopping board thoroughly before touching other foods, or your baby
• Don't store wholegrain flour at room temperature too long, as its fats could go rancid

Keep work surfaces thoroughly clean and never allow pets to climb on them. Ideally, use a disposable cloth that you replace each day. Alternatively, use a cloth or sponge and microwave it on high for 60 seconds each day; pop it in the dishwasher with the dishes on a hot cycle; or put a cloth or sponge in bleach or disinfectant solution for 30 minutes a day.

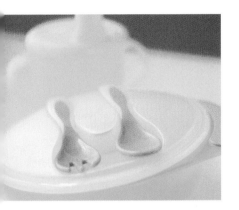

KEEPING FEEDING EQUIPMENT CLEAN

Sterilise bottles, caps, teats and bottle brushes each time you use them, whatever your child's age. Otherwise bacteria readily breed in the traces of milk or other drinks. There's no need to sterilise spoons, bowls, plates and cups used when feeding babies with solids, as long as you wash them thoroughly.

PREPARING FOOD

The way you prepare and cook your family's food can have a significant effect on its nutritional value.

VEGETABLES AND FRUIT

Wash vegetables and fruit before eating them raw or cooking them unpeeled, to remove dirt and pesticide residues. Peel carrots and other root vegetables unless they're organic. Citrus fruit rind is often waxed to make it look shiny. If you want to grate the rind or liquidize the whole fruit, buy unwaxed fruit. If unobtainable, wash off the wax with really hot, soapy water. Peel vegetables and fruit immediately before serving; otherwise enzymes will react with the air to turn the cut surface brown, and they'll lose vitamin C. Use the outer leaves of Brussels sprouts, cauliflower leaf stems and other trimmings in casseroles and soups for extra flavour, bulk and nutrients.

Cook vegetables and fruit as lightly as possible so they taste better and retain more vitamin C, vitamin B12 and folic acid. Use the cooking water to make soup, gravy or sauce, or to moisten your baby's purées.

MEAT

Select lean cuts of meat and trim off most of the obvious fat before cooking.

FRYING

Concentrated fats and oils form part of a balanced diet only if used in moderation, so use the minimum for frying. Favour polyunsaturated oils, such as sunflower, rapeseed (canola) and corn oil, and mono-unsaturated olive oil. Don't burn fried food because very high temperatures encourage the formation of unhealthy 'trans' fats. Deep-frying can make foods very fatty, and is the least safe method of cooking when children are around.

SALT AND SALTY FOODS

Try to avoid adding salt as you cook – and never do so for under-ones. Instead of using salt, add herbs and hints of spices to give more flavour to foods when necessary. If babies have too much salt their kidneys might, at worst, be unable to get rid of it, which could make them dangerously ill. The culprit in salt is the mineral sodium – so under-ones should also avoid non-salty foods that are rich in sodium.

Common salty or sodium-rich foods are: bacon, kippers and other smoked food; sausages; paté; stock cubes; yeast extracts, such as Marmite; soy sauce; tomato ketchup; many chutneys and pickled foods; many 'ready' meals – including soups, cook-chilled and frozen meals; many canned vegetables; bicarbonate of soda and baking powder.

ADDING SUGAR

Try to avoid adding sugar to food. Think twice about sprinkling sugar on cereals or fruit for your children, or adding it to their tea. Too much added sugar isn't good for them, especially for their teeth (see page 31). The recipes in this book have been devised to keep the level of added sugar low. Try reducing the sugar in other recipes for cakes, biscuits and desserts by up to half. Instead, enrich them with natural sweetness from fresh or dried fruit, or vegetables such as carrots, beetroot and sweet potato. Remember to clean your child's teeth after foods containing sugar.

USING HERBS AND SPICES

The wider the range of flavours young children experience in the first few years – and the first year in particular – the wider the range of foods they are likely to find acceptable later. So it's a good idea to introduce them to spicy and other interesting flavours early on, though these shouldn't be strong at first. I did this gradually with mine, for example, by adding only hints of herbs and spices at first, and gradually increasing the amount as they met with approval.

A HEALTHY BODY WEIGHT

It's normal for many young children to be a little plump. A few, though, are too plump. And a few are too thin. You'll probably know if this is so, but if necessary a doctor can plot your child's weight on a chart. It's only if the weight is very high or low – or if it's fast heading that way – that you need be concerned.

Young children naturally tend to become more streamlined as they approach 5 years. However, older children are more likely to be heavy if they have an overweight parent – even more so if both parents are overweight. So if your child has a weight problem and you do too, it's wise to do something about yourself before focusing on your child. Your example of healthy eating and exercising, and managing stress without comfort eating, may do more to help your overweight child than anything else.

OVERWEIGHT

Children who are overweight may well lose their excess kilos (or pounds) as they grow. However, without being 'fattist', it really is best from a health – and, perhaps, happiness – point of view for a child not to be too overweight. It can be very tiring, and plump schoolchildren are often teased, bullied or left out of peer group activities. But the main health hazard is that it makes children more likely to be obese as adults. And that encourages many health problems, including heart disease, back pain, arthritis and some cancers. Experts say children are getting fatter. So it's up to parents to stop this happening. A child may become overweight because they are:
• Exercising too little
• Eating a poor diet – often with too much high-GI food (see Tiredness, page 31)
• Eating too much
• Eating to deal with stress
• Suffering from a medical condition, though this is unlikely
What to do: Simply make sure you offer a healthy balanced diet, regular meals and, most important, encourage daily exercise. Then slowly, as your child grows, the weight will gradually enter the healthy range. Don't start a weight-reducing diet unless it is advised – and supervised – by a doctor.

UNDERWEIGHT

Being underweight is far less likely in developed countries than being overweight, but a child may become too light if they eat too little, take too much exercise, feel very stressed, or have a medical condition, such as an overactive thyroid gland or worms.

MANAGING FUSSY EATERS

Children who eat sitting at the table with other people are more likely to eat well and with less fuss, partly perhaps because they don't feel all the attention is focused on them. Try to encourage calm, unrushed mealtimes, because this helps digestive juices to flow, and this, in turn, helps the body absorb nutrients. Sharing mealtimes also gives everyone a chance to talk and be listened to. Fussiness can show up in one of several ways:

DISLIKE OF LUMPY FOODS

The most common reason for babies disliking lumpy foods is that they've become too used to smooth purées. First tastes of foods other than milk must be puréed smoothly, but after a few weeks, introduce slightly less smooth purées. Mashing foods that are soft enough – such as cooked carrots and squash – is a good way of doing this, because it doesn't get food as smooth as blending or sieving. Alternatively, whizz the food in the blender for a shorter time. Babies who have been given purées from around 4 months can start coping with slightly lumpy food from around 6 months.

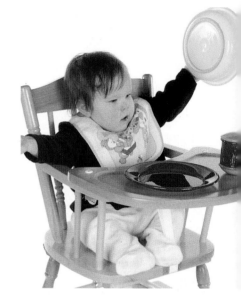

Some babies dislike lumpy foods because these are introduced too early, or they are put off by choking on a lump. Be guided by your baby; if he or she is coping brilliantly with smoothly puréed food, offer slightly less smooth food for a week or two, then gradually introduce slightly lumpy food, and progress to bigger lumps. If at any stage he or she splutters or protests over lumpy food, make it a little bit smoother next time.

PLAYING WITH FOOD

Young children play with food for a number of reasons. They may not be hungry, perhaps because they've been drinking a lot, or eating too many snacks. Alternatively, they may be ill or upset. If you think your child is unwell, get help, if necessary. If you think the child is upset, encourage him or her – if old enough – to talk about it, or give a cuddle, or simply a bit of space to recover.

PICKINESS

While it's wise to offer a little of everything, it isn't advisable to make a fuss if a young child doesn't eat something, as this could encourage longer lasting problems. Also, the food may genuinely make the child unwell. Be guided by your instinct and knowledge of your child's individual likes and dislikes.

Serve only a tiny amount of any food your child isn't keen on, and say nothing if it's left. Offer it again every so often; one day you may be surprised to find it gone. Don't get anxious about how much your child does or doesn't eat, as your child will detect this. Sometimes pickiness has to do with disliking a food's smell, taste, appearance or texture; preparing it in a different way can make all the difference. Children are more likely to be picky about certain foods:

If your child won't eat vegetables: They may dislike the taste or texture. Don't insist that they eat them, but try the following:
• Introduce many different varieties, including beans and lentils.
• Present vegetables in various ways. If your child doesn't like cooked carrots try raw carrot sticks, for example.
• Disguise vegetables among other foods. For example, blend the sauce for Autumn Pasta (see page 45), or the parsnip in Shark Soup (see page 67) so pieces of vegetable aren't visible.
• Offer more fruits instead.

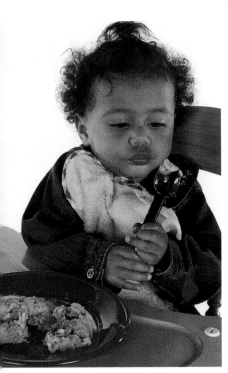

If your child won't eat fruit: Don't force the issue, because they may well develop a liking for it when they are older. Try the following positive steps:
• Provide plenty of variety. Offer fruits of different colours in different guises: raw, dried and cooked; chopped, puréed, and cut into sticks as finger foods.
• Try disguising fruit: for example, hide strawberries in Pink Tubby Custard (see page 103), blend the sauce with the rice in Rice Pudding with Fruit Sauce (see page 106), or make a banana shake (see Gotta Lotta Bottle, see page 77).
• Offer more vegetables instead.

If your child won't drink milk: Seek advice from a dietician or doctor and consider other ways of giving the nutrients it provides:
• Hide it in other foods, such as Baked Plum Custard (see page 102) or Drop Scones (see page 37), or blend some into soup.
• Give cheese, yogurt and fromage frais instead.
• Use non-dairy alternatives to provide protein, fat and calcium.

If your child won't eat meat: It is probably because they find it hard to chew, dislike the taste of its fat, or get small bits of meat stuck between their teeth. Try the following:
• Prepare meat differently, perhaps by mincing it very finely, or cooking it until it's softer.
• Serve different meats; try giving cold meat; or offer unusual combinations, such as Bacon-wrapped Prunes (see page 141).
• Give other proteins, such as eggs, as in Pocket Omelette (see page 35); fish, as in Salmon & Pasta Salad (see page 79); and beans, as in Every Flavour Beans (see page 69).

FOOD REFUSAL

It's disconcerting when a baby or young child refuses to eat what you've prepared. Don't take it personally, but try to work out what's going on. Your baby might be more in need of a drink than food, or he or she might be too hot or cold. Alternatively, a cold wet nappy, or a sore bottom, could be distracting the baby's attention from food. Or your baby may be teething – as a tooth pushes up, it makes the gum itchy and sore. Other causes include teasing by a sibling; remembering that the last meal was too hot; having a cold, sore throat or other infection; or simply testing your limits. In some children, food refusal is a sign of underlying anger, loneliness, frustration, or even depression. If you suspect any of these, discuss it with your doctor.

LACK OF APPETITE

Sometimes a child doesn't feel like eating. If a schoolchild won't eat breakfast, you won't want them to go all morning on an empty tummy, so provide a healthy 'break' your child likes, such as a banana. Sometimes the problem is social or emotional. If your child won't eat school lunch, for example, it may be because they aren't sitting with a friend. Or it could indicate unhappiness or insecurity about something or someone at home or school. A little detective work can work wonders and a child who knows you will help sort things out will probably eat well again quite soon. A loss of appetite can indicate that something is medically wrong, so if it continues, ask for your doctor's advice.

FOODS FOR COMMON AILMENTS

Using food as a medicine isn't a new idea – many traditional remedies involve giving specific foods for particular ailments. For example, homemade lemon barley water and chicken soup are recommended to relieve a cold. And many old wives' tales learnt from our parents, like 'an apple a day keeps the doctor away' focus on using everyday foods to prevent and treat common ailments. Kitchen-based home cures are pleasant to use and I have found many to be very successful. In recent years, researchers have found a scientific basis for many of these traditional remedies.

You can help prevent and treat certain common health problems simply by encouraging your children to eat more of certain foods, or less of others, as outlined here.

GENERAL ADVICE
• Do seek medical help for any new or unfamiliar ailment that is serious or doesn't soon get better.
• Do continue to use other remedies, medicines or therapies.
• Don't worry if your child doesn't want to eat something different. If you get stressed, your child will get upset too, which might hinder recovery. So don't insist unless your doctor explains that you must.
• Don't make any major changes to your child's diet – such as cutting out milk or wheat – without seeking advice from your doctor or other competent health professional, or your child could go short of vital protein, fats, vitamins, calcium or calories.

ANAEMIA
Help to prevent and treat iron-deficiency anaemia by giving more foods that are rich in iron, vitamin C and copper. Try giving liver, fish, shellfish, cheese, egg yolk, green vegetables, apricots, cherries and figs. Iron-rich recipes include Magic Mince (see page 90), Every Flavour Beans (see page 69), and Baked Plum Custard (see page 102). Give your child some orange juice to drink with meals, as vitamin C helps the body to absorb iron, but avoid tea or cola.

ANXIETY
If your child seems anxious or depressed, yet there's nothing obviously wrong, offer more foods that are rich in vitamins B, C and E, calcium, magnesium, omega-3 fats, and an amino acid called tryptophan. The best way of getting tryptophan to the brain, where it's needed, is by having carbohydrate snacks such as bananas, Banana Teabread (see page 129) or Flapjacks (see page 128) mid-morning and at teatime. Avoid giving too much meat, and drinks that contain caffeine, such as tea and cola. Help to keep your child's blood-sugar level from dipping by including some foods with a low 'glycaemic index' (see Tiredness, page 31) with each meal, and avoid long gaps between meals.

ASTHMA
To help prevent allergic asthma, offer more foods that are rich in beta-carotene; vitamins B, C and E; magnesium, selenium and zinc; and plant pigments. Onions, berries, oily fish and buckwheat are especially useful. Encourage a good balance of essential fats by cooking with rapeseed (canola), olive or walnut oil, rather than corn or sunflower oil, and offering green leafy vegetables, beans, sweet potatoes and wholegrain foods.

BED-WETTING
Never let your child go thirsty, but don't encourage them to drink a lot in the evening. Make sure they don't have drinks that contain caffeine, such as cola or tea, after 4 pm. Also, try to avoid foods with added colourings, as these sometimes irritate the bladder and encourage accidents at night. Foods containing oxalates, such as spinach, strawberries and rhubarb, can have the same effect, though not if eaten with calcium-rich foods. Recipes such as Pink Tubby Custard (see page 103) and Spinach & Ricotta Puff Pie (see page 93) are therefore fine.

BEHAVIOUR PROBLEMS
Sometimes anxiety or tiredness triggers behaviour problems (see advice under these entries). Offer foods rich in vitamins B and E; calcium, magnesium and zinc; omega-3 fats; and the amino acid called tryptophan (see Anxiety). Have a good balance of essential fats and avoid too much animal protein. Cut down on refined carbohydrates, favouring unrefined ones, such as oats, as in Baby Bear's Big Breakfast (see page 34). Iron-deficiency anaemia or food sensitivity is occasionally to blame; if you suspect one of these, see the doctor.

COLD SORES
Follow the general advice under Infection. Favour foods that are rich in the amino acid called lysine, and cut down on foods that are rich in arginine – another amino acid. You can do this by offering more potatoes, while cutting back on foods containing wheat or other grain, seeds and chocolate.

COLDS AND FLU

See the advice under Infection, and offer plenty to drink. A homemade lemon drink is ideal: Pour boiling water over a sliced lemon and sweeten with a little honey for children over one; leave until cool enough for your child to drink. Homemade Chicken Soup (see page 68) is a proven remedy; it speeds the flow of nasal mucus, boosts immunity and counteracts inflammation in the nose.

COLIC

Food sensitivity, Indigestion or Constipation may be the cause of colic; refer to the advice under the appropriate entry if you think it is relevant. If your breastfed baby tends to be colicky, make sure you eat something nutritious between breastfeeds and, if you feel stressed, follow the advice under Anxiety for yourself.

CONSTIPATION

Try to prevent constipation but if it occurs, deal with it promptly. The pain when a hard, bulky bowel motion is eventually passed may make your child put off going the next time for as long as possible, which makes things worse. Encourage your child to drink plenty of fluids; the urine should be very pale yellow. Offer plenty of foods that are naturally rich in fibre, such as Bubble & Squeak (see page 59) and Every Flavour Beans (see page 69). Give less white bread and other food made with refined white flour. Don't give young children foods that contain concentrated bran, such as bran breakfast cereals, as these fill them up and may reduce their appetite for other foods they need.

DIARRHOEA

Don't confuse this with the normal, frequent loose bowel motions of a breastfed baby. And don't be alarmed when you see bits of food such as seeds in an older baby's or young toddler's motions. This is sometimes called 'toddler diarrhoea', but is perfectly normal. Sometimes diarrhoea occurs when softer bowel motions leak around a hard motion in a constipated child (see Constipation). See also Gastroenteritis and Lactose intolerance.

DRY SKIN

Offer more foods that are rich in beta-carotene, vitamins C and E, zinc and omega-3 fats. Beta-carotene is particularly important, and good recipes for boosting this vitamin include Sage & Squash Gnocchi (see page 74), Autumn Pasta (see page 45) and Frittata (see page 58).

ECZEMA

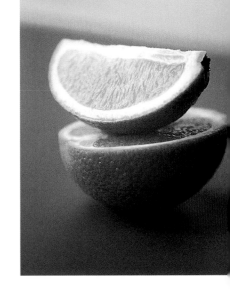

Full breastfeeding for the first 4 to 6 months may delay the onset of eczema or at least, if it does appear, make it less severe. For babies under one with allergy in the family, removing certain foods from the diet and from the diet of breastfeeding mothers, can reduce the risk of eczema significantly (see page 19). Once eczema develops, changing the diet usually makes no difference. But if your child's eczema always worsens after one particular food, consider eliminating it for 3 months to see if there is an improvement, but take guidance from a doctor or dietician on maintaining a balanced diet without this food.

To help soothe inflamed skin, offer more foods that are rich in vitamins A and B, zinc and omega-3 fats; and help counter allergy with foods rich in beta-carotene, vitamins C and E, selenium and plant pigments. Celery, citrus fruit, parsley, parsnips and watercress may also help because they contain substances called psoralens that boost the healing action of sunlight on eczematous skin.

FITS

The frequency of some types of seizure can be reduced by eating foods that are rich in vitamins B6 and E, copper (in liver, shellfish, avocados, nuts, olive, beans, peas, wholegrain foods), magnesium and selenium. Food sensitivity can very occasionally trigger fits; if you suspect this, seek your doctor's advice.

FOOD SENSITIVITY

If you suspect your child may be sensitive to a particular food, seek medical advice. Food allergy is one sort of food sensitivity; it is most likely to occur if there is a family history of allergy (see page 19 for advice). Boost your child's immunity with more foods that are rich in beta-carotene, vitamins C and E, selenium, zinc and omega-3 fats. See also Allergy, Gluten intolerance and Lactose intolerance.

FUNGAL SKIN AND NAIL INFECTIONS

Refer to the advice under Infection. In addition, avoid giving your child too many foods which contain added sugar or white flour.

GASTROENTERITIS

Treat diarrhoea and vomiting by offering plenty of fluids, such as water, well diluted fruit juice, weak tea or vegetable broth. If it lasts longer than a day, give drinks made from oral rehydration salts (from a pharmacy), or make your own by dissolving 1 level teaspoon of salt and 8 level teaspoons of sugar in 1 litre (1¾ pints) of water. Once your child can keep food down, offer easily digested food such as brown rice, ripe bananas and live yogurt. Also, see Infection. Get medical help should any of the following apply: a child can't keep any fluids down; a very young child has severe diarrhoea for 12 hours or mild diarrhoea for 24 hours; an over-five has severe diarrhoea for 48 hours or mild diarrhoea for 72 hours; a child's motions contain blood.

GLUTEN SENSITIVITY

Gluten is a protein found in wheat, barley, rye, and often oats. Whole oats don't contain gluten, but most oatmeal is contaminated with up to 15% of wheat flour during milling. Sensitivity to gluten can lead to coeliac disease, with tummy ache, wind and weight loss, due to poor absorption of nutrients. It can also trigger a wide variety of other symptoms. The risk of developing coeliac disease is reduced if the above foods aren't given to babies under 6 months.

If your child has a proven gluten sensitivity, avoid these grains entirely. Instead, offer corn, as in Traffic Lights (see page 94) and Sweetcorn Griddle Cakes (see page 76); and rice, as in Rice Pudding with Fruit Sauce (see page 106). Buckwheat, millet and sorghum are other non-gluten alternatives.

'GROWING PAINS'

Up to one in five children between the ages of 4 and 12 sometimes experiences cramps or other muscle pains, typically in the legs. The usual culprit is swelling of a muscle as a consequence of being very active, or exercising on a hard surface like tarmac. Help prevent these pains by giving more foods that are rich in calcium, magnesium, potassium, zinc, vitamins C and E, and omega-3 fats.

HAY FEVER

Follow the advice under Asthma for counteracting allergy and boosting immunity. Give your child 2 teaspoons of locally produced honeycomb a day for the 2 months before you expect hay fever to begin. Honey isn't suitable for under-ones, but they don't get hay fever.

HEADACHE

If you think your child's headache is caused by tension, see Anxiety. To help prevent migraine, try giving more foods that are rich in omega-3 fats. During an attack, try offering ginger tea once or twice a day. If you suspect that food sensitivity may be to blame, see your doctor.

INDIGESTION

Help prevent this by avoiding rushed meals. Start main meals with a little salad – the fibre will line the stomach and help protect it from any excess of acid. Offer more foods that are rich in vitamins B, C and zinc, and slightly bitter foods such as lettuce, cabbage, watercress, chicory, turnips and rosemary. Try adding a little vinegar or lemon juice to meat and fish. Keep meals relatively small. Never force a child to eat, and get medical help if you suspect a food sensitivity. Treat indigestion by offering some pineapple or papaya, or some ginger, chamomile or mint tea.

INFECTION

Boost immunity by giving your child more foods that are rich in beta-carotene, vitamins C and E, selenium, zinc and plant pigments. Many herbs are useful in boosting immunity as well as easing the symptoms of infections, including oregano with its potent antioxidants, and sage which contains a natural antiseptic called thujone. Give your child enough drinks to keep urine pale yellow. Garlic has anti-viral and anti-bacterial properties; onions are good too, especially eaten raw. Barley also contains anti-viral agents called protease inhibitors; try giving Barley Pot (see page 91), or homemade lemon barley water – boil pot barley until soft, then cool and add sliced lemon to the strained barley water).

LACTOSE INTOLERANCE

Tummy ache, wind and diarrhoea sometimes result from the poor digestion of lactose (milk sugar). This can happen temporarily after gastroenteritis, but in some older children digesting more than 300 ml (½ pint) of milk at a time is a permanent problem. The cause is a lack of lactase, the enzyme in the gut that digests lactose. Discuss with your doctor whether milk should be limited or avoided if your child has persistent diarrhoea. For older children with proven permanent lactose intolerance, either limit milk (with guidance on alternative foods from a doctor or dietician), or add a lactase supplement (available from the pharmacy) to milk before using it. Yogurt is usually well digested because its bacteria produce lactase.

MOUTH ULCERS

Encourage your child to eat slowly so as to avoid biting the insides of their cheeks. Avoid giving sugary or acidic foods and drinks, and avoid boiled sweets containing E100-155 colourings. Mouth ulcers may indicate a food sensitivity problem, such as gluten sensitivity. Also, refer to the advice under Infection.

NAIL PROBLEMS

If your child's nails are splitting or breaking, try to give more foods that are rich in protein, calcium, magnesium, zinc and essential fats. Iron-deficiency anaemia can cause nail problems, too (see Anaemia). See also Fungal skin and nail infections.

PSORIASIS

Offer more foods that are rich in folic acid, selenium, zinc and essential fats. Help counteract underlying inflammation by using olive oil in salad dressings and for cooking; giving oily fish, such as Coconut Mackerel with Sweet Potato (see page 82); and spicing food with turmeric. Celery, citrus fruit, figs, parsley, parsnips and watercress may also help. These foods are rich in psoralens, which encourage the healing action of sunlight on skin affected by psoriasis. Sometimes having less meat helps, and occasionally gluten sensitivity is to blame (see entry).

SLEEP PROBLEMS

Make your child's last meal relatively early in the evening. It should be light, carbohydrate-rich, and cheese-free. Don't give tea, cocoa or cola after 4 pm. Favour foods that are rich in vitamin B, calcium, magnesium and zinc. Lettuce, rosemary and thyme are reputed to aid sleep.

TIREDNESS

Offer more foods that are rich in vitamins B, C and E, folic acid, iron, magnesium, potassium and omega-3 fats. Cut down on refined carbohydrates, such as bread, biscuits and cake made with white flour. Favour foods with a low glycaemic index (low GI); these raise the blood sugar only slowly, which is preferable. They include proteins, dairy foods, nuts, oats, most vegetables (but not potatoes, broad beans or canned beans), and many fruits (but not bananas, grapes, pineapple or watermelon).

Offer foods with a moderately high GI (canned beans, peas, oranges, biscuits, pasta, sweetcorn, potato, sugar and chocolate) together with low GI-foods to help counteract a rapid rise in blood sugar. Offer high-GI foods (bananas, raisins, beetroot, broad beans, carrots, corn chips, corn flakes, white bread, puffed or shredded wheat, rice, honey, low-fat ice cream) in very small amounts, and ideally always with some low-GI food.

TOOTH DECAY

Never put sugary fluid like squash or other sugared fruit drinks in or on a dummy, because this will bathe the mouth and encourage tooth decay to begin before the first tooth emerges. Ideally, avoid foods containing added sugar for under-ones; but if they do have them, clean their teeth and gums afterwards.

Limit foods and drinks that contain added sugar to mealtimes, as the lengthy chewing that goes on during a proper meal increases saliva flow, which washes most of the sugar away. Brushing teeth, eating fibrous food (such as raw celery or carrot), or swishing water around the mouth also gets rid of traces of sugar. If this isn't done, mouth bacteria break them down. This releases acid, which encourages tooth decay. It's possible to neutralise acid after a sugary meal by eating cheese or nuts. Clean a baby's or young child's teeth yourself, and use a sterile cloth to wipe the gums of a baby who hasn't any teeth.

Water and milk are the best between-meal drinks, but don't give sugary drinks such as squash and cola, or fizzy drinks. Fruit juice isn't ideal between meals either. Fruit contains natural fruit sugars. If you eat fruit between meals, the necessary chewing (except for soft fruit like bananas) stimulates saliva production, which washes away fruit sugar – this doesn't happen with fruit juice. If children do have sugary or fizzy drinks between meals, give them a straw; this directs the fluid to the back of the mouth rather than over the teeth.

Strengthen your child's teeth by giving more foods that are rich in calcium, magnesium and other minerals. Teach older children how to floss their teeth.

WIND

Encourage relaxed mealtimes. If wind is a particular problem, you may wish to adapt meals to counteract it. Eating fruit after fatty foods may increase wind, because fats take a relatively long time to be digested, which encourages the fermentation of fruit sugars in the gut. The same applies to eating fruit with refined carbohydrates, as these are slow to pass through the bowel, giving more time for fruit sugar to ferment. Sulphur-containing foods such as eggs can cause offensive wind. If you are breastfeeding, you may find that eating certain foods, such as onions and cabbage, encourages your baby to be windy.

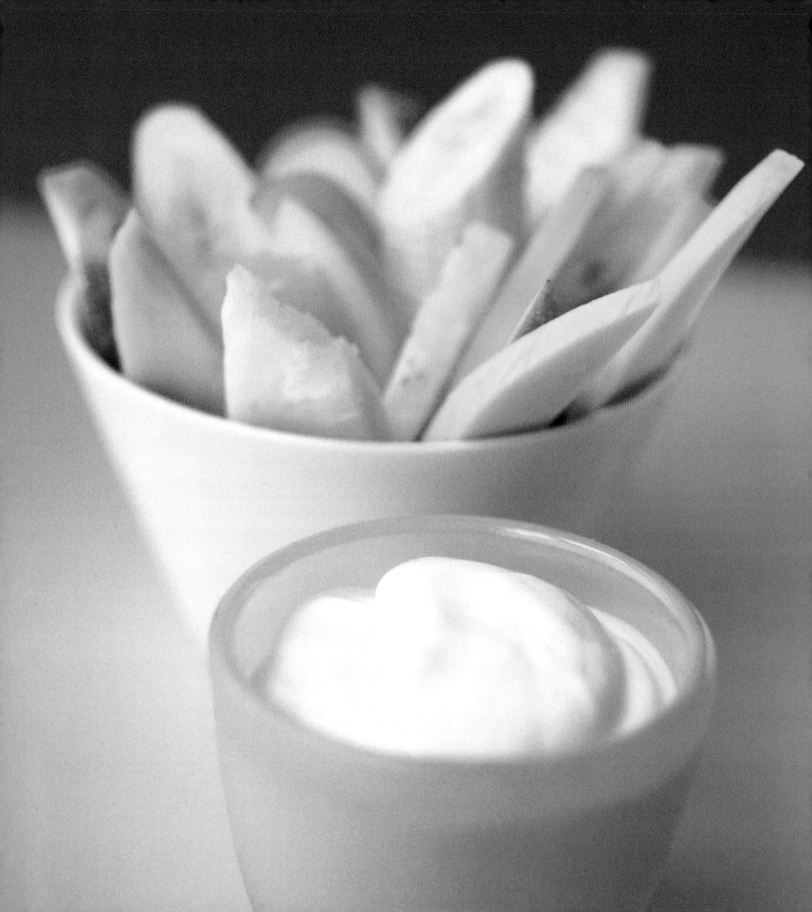

Start the day right

I recommend that you and your family 'breakfast like kings', for starting the day with a good well-balanced meal has many benefits. It boosts the metabolism, provides energy to last the morning, and gives your body cells the mix of nutrients they need to work to their full potential. So make sure everyone finds time to sit down and break their overnight fast, then you will all be ready for whatever the day may bring.

FINGER FRUITS & YOGURT

Nothing could be more appealing to young children than dipping fresh fruit into creamy, tangy yogurt. Ring the changes with fresh strawberries or raspberries, or sweet, juicy pineapple when you have time to prepare it.

1-2 apples or pears

1 orange

1 mango

½ small pineapple (optional)

1-2 bananas

475 ml (16 fl oz) natural, creamy 'bio' yogurt

a little muscovado sugar, to taste (optional)

Quarter and core the apples or pears, peel if preferred and cut into long slices. Peel the orange and divide into segments. Peel the mango and cut the flesh away from the stone, then slice. Peel the pineapple and slice into rings or sticks, cutting out the central core. Peel and halve the bananas.

Arrange the 'finger fruits' on individual plates with a small bowl of yogurt. Serve the muscovado sugar separately.

BONUS POINTS
• Most yogurts – except 'long-life' (UHT, pasteurised or sterilised) types – contain some live bacteria, but 'bio' yogurts contain the most. There's some evidence that yogurts with over a million live bacteria per gram have several health benefits, such as helping prevent diarrhoea.
• Children and adults with lactose intolerance (tummy-ache, wind or diarrhoea from milk sugar) can often digest yogurt.

OKAY FOR UNDER-ONES?
4-6 months Omit yogurt. Blend apples, pears, mangoes or pineapple with a little milk, or mash banana with a little milk.
6-12 months Make sure you buy unsweetened yogurt and omit the muscovado sugar. Blend or mash the fruit with yogurt until your baby is able to chew, then cut it into small pieces or sticks that they can hold.

• Give under-twos whole-fat yogurt; 2-5 year olds can have either whole- or half-fat yogurt; anyone over 5 years can have whole-, half or low-fat yogurt.

BABY BEAR'S BIG BREAKFAST

A bowl of comforting, warm porridge makes a wonderfully sustaining breakfast which can be sweetened and enhanced to taste with fresh, cooked or dried fruit, or a little honey or jam.

125 g (4 oz) quick-cook porridge oats

1.2 litres (2 pints) milk or water (see tip box)

To serve:

4 ripe bananas, thinly sliced, or 75 g (3 oz) sultanas or chopped dried dates, or 250 g (8 oz) stewed apricots

a little honey or reduced-sugar apricot or cherry jam (optional)

Put the porridge oats and milk (or water) in a large saucepan and bring to the boil. Simmer, stirring occasionally, for about 5 minutes, until thickened.

Divide the porridge between serving bowls. Add fruit (or jam or honey) to babies and toddlers portions. Let older children and adults flavour their portions to taste.

BONUS POINTS

• Oats contain thiamine and other important B vitamins (for energy, calmness and good vision); calcium (for healthy nerves, and strong bones and teeth); and iron (for transporting oxygen in the blood).
• Porridge provides 'slow-release' carbohydrate (that steadies the blood-sugar level) and soluble fibre (that lowers the blood cholesterol level).

OKAY FOR UNDER-ONES?

4-6 months Not suitable. Instead, give some banana mashed with a little milk, or some puréed and sieved stewed apricots.
6-12 months Make the porridge with whole milk. Don't give honey. Mash the bananas well, or purée sultanas, dates or apricots. When your baby can cope with lumps, cut the fruit into small pieces or sticks. Clean your baby's teeth and gums afterwards.

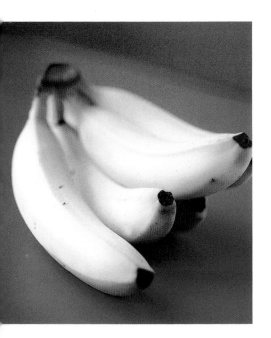

• Porridge made with milk rather than water is creamier and sweeter, although some children prefer milk-free porridge. If your family includes any children under 2 years use full-fat milk; otherwise use semi-skimmed milk.

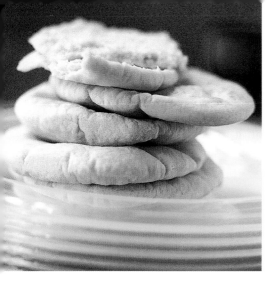

POCKET OMELETTE

Stuff a pitta bread with a folded-over vegetable omelette and you have the perfect fortifying breakfast. No knives or forks are required – children can simply pick up their breakfast and munch! The soft, moist omelette contrasts well with the firmer texture of pitta bread, and next time you can ring the changes by varying the vegetables. You will need a frying pan that is suitable for use under the grill.

1 tablespoon canola (rapeseed), olive or walnut oil

2 carrots, grated, or 4 tomatoes, chopped, or 125 g (4 oz) cabbage, spinach or pak choi, chopped

6 eggs

4 pitta breads

salt (optional) and black pepper

Heat the oil in a large frying pan, add the carrots, tomatoes, cabbage or other greens, and cook for 2-3 minutes until they start to soften.

Meanwhile, break the eggs into a bowl, add a little salt (if using) and pepper, and beat with a fork until smooth and frothy.

Pour the egg mixture over the vegetables in the pan, and quickly mix together using a wooden spoon. Cook, without stirring, until the top is just set, lifting the edges of the omelette to allow the uncooked egg to run underneath. Pop under the grill to lightly brown the top.

Warm the pitta breads briefly in the toaster or microwave, or under the grill; do not overheat or they will become brittle. Open each along one long side, using a sharp knife or scissors.

Cut the omelette into wedges, roll each one loosely, then place in an opened pitta pocket. Serve hot or warm, with homemade tomato ketchup (see page 36) if you like.

BONUS POINTS
• This is a good way of getting children who are reluctant to eat vegetables accustomed to their flavour, and helps everyone towards the recommended five helpings of vegetables and fruit a day.
• The chlorophyll pigment in green leafy vegetables is a good source of magnesium, a mineral we all need to keep our bones and teeth strong.

OKAY FOR UNDER-ONES?
Omit salt and let older people add it separately.
4-6 months Not suitable. Instead, steam or boil some carrots and purée with a little milk or cooking water.
6-9 months Blend the food with a little milk or water. Or, when your baby can chew, cut into small pieces and add a little milk or water to soften the bread. Some babies like to hold a piece of pitta bread.
9-12 months Cut up small, or give your baby a piece to hold.

• Small pitta breads or 'picnic pittas' are available from most supermarkets and are useful for those with smaller appetites; alternatively, ordinary pitta breads can be halved and filled widthways.
• Add a further tang to the omelette by sprinkling the top with 25-50 g (1-2 oz) grated cheese before popping under the grill.

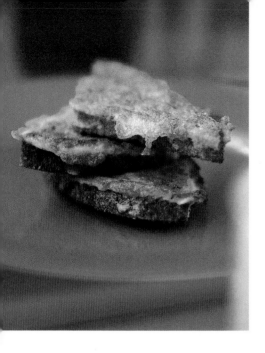

EGGY BREAD

Golden eggy bread is popular with kids of all ages. It can be served either savoury or sweet, and is a nutritious way to start the day.

Break the eggs into a bowl, add a small pinch of salt (if using) and pepper, and beat with a fork until smooth.

Heat the oil in a large non-stick frying pan. Dip a piece of bread in the egg mixture to coat, then add to the pan; repeat with the other pieces of bread. Pour any leftover egg into the pan. Cook until lightly browned underneath.

Separate the pieces of eggy bread if necessary, then turn them over and cook until golden brown on the other side. Drain on kitchen paper.

Serve hot or warm, with grilled tomatoes or homemade tomato ketchup (see below). Alternatively, serve with a little reduced-sugar jam, honey or marmalade.

BONUS POINT
Both the oil and eggs provide alpha-linolenic acid, the essential omega-3 fatty acid that helps counter infection, allergy and inflammation.

OKAY FOR UNDER-ONES?
Omit the salt (others can add it separately). Omit the honey too.
4-6 months Not suitable. See pages 16-19 for other ideas.
6-9 months Blend the eggy bread with a little milk or water or, once your baby can chew, cut into small pieces and soften by soaking in a little milk or water for a few minutes.
9-12 months Either cut up small, or give your baby a piece to hold.

HOMEMADE TOMATO KETCHUP
Chop 8 tomatoes and put into a small pan with 2 teaspoons tomato purée, 2 tablespoons water, ½-1 crushed garlic clove, ½-1 teaspoon chopped fresh basil (or a pinch of dried), and a sprinkling of black pepper. Cook, stirring, for 5 minutes. Cool, then blend until smooth; pass through a sieve to remove skins and seeds. Store the ketchup in a screw-top jar in the refrigerator for up to 3 days, or freeze in convenient portions in ice-cube trays and defrost at room temperature as required.

4 eggs
1 tablespoon canola (rapeseed), olive or walnut oil
4 slices wholemeal bread, cut into quarters or shapes
salt (optional) and black pepper

• If your children don't like wholemeal, use brown or fibre-enriched white bread, adding a little more pepper or a pinch of dried oregano to the beaten egg, to enhance the flavour.

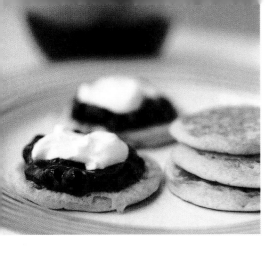

DROP SCONES

These delicious little flat scones are quick and easy to cook and unbelievably moreish, especially with a topping to tantalise the tastebuds. You can either whisk up the batter first thing in the morning, or do so the night before and let it rest overnight in the refrigerator.

250 g (8 oz) plain flour
1 teaspoon bicarbonate of soda
2 teaspoons cream of tartar
1 tablespoon caster sugar
2 eggs
1 teaspoon sunflower or corn oil
300 ml (½ pint) milk
unsalted butter, for frying

Topping (optional):
75 g (3 oz) blueberries
2 tablespoons water
75 g (3 oz) Greek yogurt

Put the flour, bicarbonate of soda, cream of tartar and sugar in a bowl and make a well in the centre. Add the eggs, oil and half of the milk to the well, and gradually incorporate the flour with a whisk. Add the remaining milk and whisk well to make a smooth batter.

For the topping (if required), put the blueberries and water in a small pan and cook gently for 2-3 minutes to soften slightly.

Melt a small knob of butter in a large non-stick frying pan. Cook the scones in batches. Drop large spoonfuls of batter into the pan from the tip of the spoon to form rounds, spacing well apart. Cook for 2-3 minutes until bubbles appear on the surface and burst, then turn them over and cook for a further 1-2 minutes until golden brown underneath. Put the scones on a clean tea towel and fold it over to keep them warm, while cooking the rest of them.

Serve the scones warm, either plain or topped with a spoonful of the blueberry compote and a dollop of yogurt.

BONUS POINTS
• A good way of giving calcium-rich milk to children who prefer not to drink it.
• The blueberry topping is a good way to obtain one of those recommended 5 daily helpings of fruit and vegetables.

OKAY FOR UNDER-ONES?
Omit the bicarbonate of soda; this will slightly alter the texture but won't spoil the taste. Clean your baby's teeth and gums after eating the scones.
4-6 months Not suitable. Instead mash blueberries with a little milk.
6-9 months Either blend a scone and its topping with a little milk or water or, once your baby can chew, cut up the scone and topping and soften with a little milk or water.
9-12 months Cut up the scone and topping, or let your baby hold a piece of it.

• Use full-fat milk for under-twos, or semi-skimmed milk if your children are all older.
• To give these scones an unusual tang use buttermilk rather than ordinary milk, reducing the cream of tartar to 1 teaspoon.
• If you haven't any bicarbonate of soda and cream of tartar, use 2 teaspoons of baking powder, and self-raising rather than plain flour.

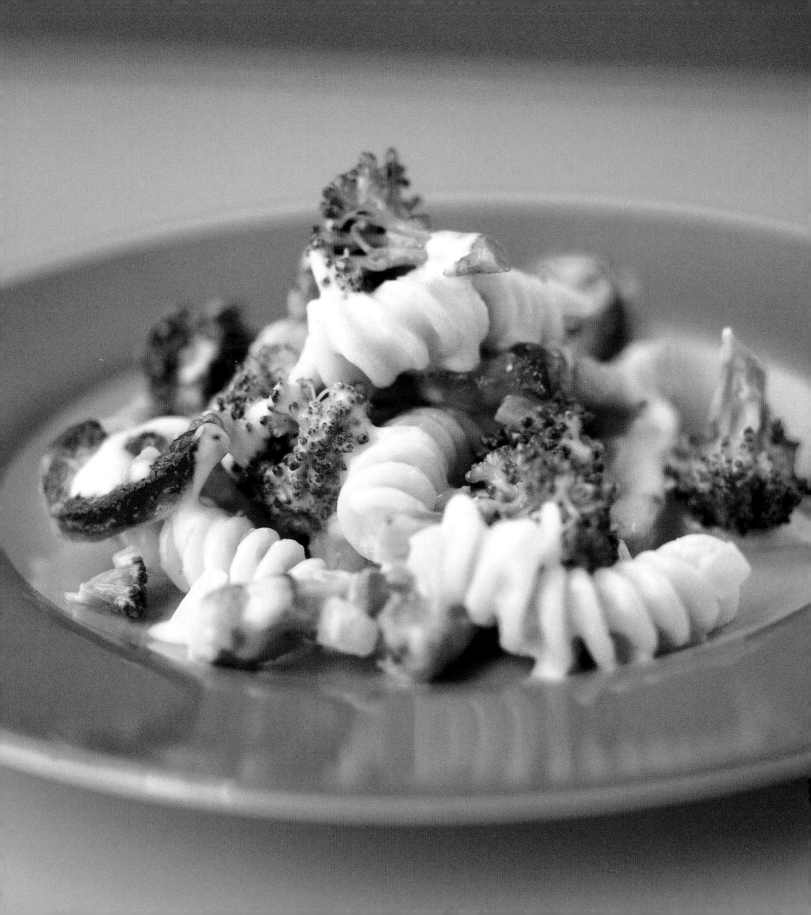

Pasta & Pizza

Pasta and pizza are great favourites with children of all ages. Available in a wide variety of shapes, sizes and colours, pasta is never dull and it's always satisfying and comforting to eat. Pizzas are equally versatile, as you can vary toppings to suit individual tastes.

CURLY COCONUT PASTA

250-375 g (8-12 oz) pasta spirals
500 g (1 lb) broccoli florets
1 tablespoon corn or rapeseed (canola) oil
1 shallot or small onion, chopped
1 garlic clove, chopped
small pinch of chilli powder (optional)
250 g (8 oz) cooked skinless chicken, cut into bite-sized pieces
4 tablespoons crème fraîche
½-1 teaspoon Dijon mustard (optional)
50 g (2 oz) creamed coconut, grated
black pepper

This combination of chicken, broccoli and pasta is popular with children and adults of all ages, partly because the coconut lends a touch of sweetness.

Cook the pasta in a large pan of boiling water for about 10 minutes until al dente – tender but firm to the bite. At the same time, cook the broccoli in a steamer over the pasta pan until just tender.

Meanwhile, heat the oil in a large frying pan, add the onion and fry for about 5 minutes until lightly browned. Add the garlic and chilli powder (if using); fry for a further 1 minute. Add the chicken, crème fraîche, mustard (if using), coconut and pepper. Heat through, stirring.

Drain the pasta spirals and stir into to the sauce. Finally, stir in the cooked broccoli florets, taking care not to break them up too much. Transfer to serving plates. Serve accompanied by a tomato salad if you like.

BONUS POINTS
• Broccoli is an excellent source of vitamin C, iron and antioxidant plant pigments called carotenes; it also contains glucosinolates that may protect against certain cancers.
• Pasta's slow-release carbohydrate helps to stabilise the blood-sugar level and prevent energy dipping 2 hours or so after a meal.

OKAY FOR UNDER-ONES?
4-6 months Not suitable. Instead, give some puréed, lightly steamed broccoli, mixed with a little milk.
6-12 months Most babies love the slightly sweet, nutty taste of this pasta dish. Omit the chilli and mustard. Blend the pasta with a little sauce. Once your baby can cope with lumps, cut the pasta up small.

• If you're not cooking for under-ones, and your family likes spicy flavours, use ½ teaspoon chilli powder and 2 teaspoons mustard.
• If you are cooking for an under-one, stir a little mustard into the pasta after removing your baby's portion; but don't add chilli at this stage, as it needs to be cooked.

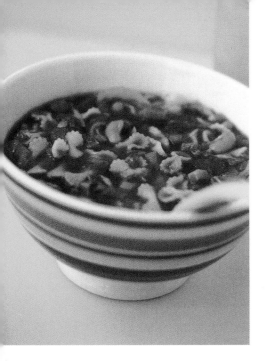

MINESTRONE

Take three Italian favourites – pasta, fresh vegetables and fruity olive oil – and you have almost all you need to prepare this fragrant, main meal soup. Minestrone is popular throughout Italy, and it is a great favourite with my family, too. Served with crusty wholemeal bread, it is substantial enough to make a meal in itself. Pastina, or tiny soup pasta, comes in a variety of shapes. Look out for alphabet pasta, numerals, dinosaurs and space paraphernalia – guaranteed toddler appeal.

1 tablespoon olive oil

1 trimmed leek or onion, finely chopped

1 garlic clove, crushed

2 carrots, finely chopped

1 celery stick, finely chopped

750 ml (1¼ pints) water

50 g (2 oz) pastina (tiny pasta shapes)

125 g (4 oz) Savoy cabbage, Brussels sprouts or other green leafy vegetable, finely shredded

425 g (14 oz) can chopped tomatoes

425 g (14 oz) can flageolet or cannellini beans

4 teaspoons chopped fresh oregano or basil (optional)

squeeze of lemon juice (optional)

salt (optional) and black pepper

Heat the oil in a large saucepan. Add the leek or onion, garlic, carrots and celery and fry gently for 4 minutes. Pour in the water and bring to the boil. Add the pasta and simmer, covered, for 5 minutes.

Add the cabbage or other greens and simmer for a further 4 minutes. Add the tomatoes, beans and pepper to taste. Stir in the herbs, lemon juice and a little salt (if using). Cook for a further 2 minutes until heated through.

Ladle the minestrone into soup bowls and serve with crusty bread.

BONUS POINTS
• A portion of minestrone provides one of the recommended 5 helpings of vegetables and fruit a day.
• Both beans and pasta provide slow-release energy that sustains children and adults for longer before they need to refuel.

OKAY FOR UNDER-ONES?
4-6 months Not suitable. Steam or boil a carrot instead, then purée with a little milk.
6-12 months Blend until your baby is old enough to chew the pasta shapes and vegetables. If the beans make your baby uncomfortably windy, leave them out next time and sprinkle the soup with a little grated cheese instead.

SPRING PASTA

You know spring is here when you first see fresh homegrown baby carrots with their leafy tops – and asparagus tips – in the shops. Baby vegetables need only the lightest of cooking, and a medley of these tossed with pasta in a creamy sauce is a real winner.

300 g (10 oz) pasta shapes

200 g (7 oz) fresh or frozen broad beans

200 g (7 oz) baby carrots, trimmed

150 g (5 oz) fine asparagus tips, trimmed and halved

2 egg yolks

6 tablespoons single cream

50 g (2 oz) Parmesan or Cheddar cheese, grated

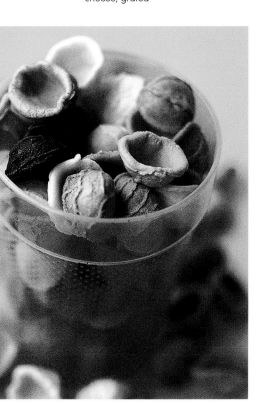

Cook the pasta in a large pan of boiling water for about 10 minutes until al dente – tender but firm to the bite.

Meanwhile steam the broad beans and carrots in a metal steamer over boiling water for 5 minutes. Add the asparagus and steam for a further 2-3 minutes until all the vegetables are just tender.

In a bowl, beat the egg yolks with the cream until evenly blended, then mix in half of the cheese.

Drain the pasta, retaining 2 tablespoons of the cooking water, and return to the pan. Add the egg mixture and vegetables and cook over a very gentle heat for 1 minute until the sauce has thickened slightly; do not overheat or the sauce might curdle.

Transfer to serving plates and serve sprinkled with the remaining cheese.

BONUS POINTS
• A good source of beta-carotene – the vitamin that's beneficial for your skin and eyes.
• Broad beans are a good source of slow-release carbohydrate, that helps keep a child's energy level high for longer.
• Egg yolk is a good source of iron.

OKAY FOR UNDER-ONES?
4-6 months Not suitable. Give your baby some steamed puréed carrot or asparagus instead.
6-12 months Purée the mixture until your baby is capable of chewing pieces of pasta and cooked vegetable – perhaps at around 8-9 months, then cut the food up very small.

PRINCESS PESTO PASTA

375-425 g (12-14 oz) wholemeal or plain
    pasta bows
1 tablespoon sunflower or corn oil
4-6 rashers of bacon, derinded and
    thinly sliced
2 onions, chopped
2 garlic cloves, crushed
375 g (12 oz) frozen peas
50 g (2 oz) pesto, preferably homemade,
    see tip box (optional)
125 ml (4 fl oz) Greek yogurt
black pepper
a little chopped fresh parsley or basil
    (optional)

• To make your own salt-free pesto,
whizz together a handful of fresh
basil leaves, 1 large garlic clove,
50 g (2 oz) pine nuts, 75 ml (3 fl oz)
olive oil, and 25 g (1 oz) grated
Parmesan cheese (or Cheddar for
under-ones).
• Keep leftover pesto refrigerated in
a screw-top jar for up to 3 days.

Peas and bacon are a particularly delicious combination. Combine them with some pretty pasta bows, Italian pesto and a sprinkling of bright green parsley or basil, and you have an easy, inexpensive meal fit for a princess.

Cook the pasta in a large pan of boiling water for about 10 minutes until al dente – tender but firm to the bite.

Meanwhile make the sauce. Heat the oil in a large frying pan, add the bacon and fry for 4-5 minutes or until lightly browned. Remove from the pan with a slotted spoon and set aside. Add the onions to the pan and fry for about 4-5 minutes, until softened but not browned. Add the garlic and fry for 1 minute.

Add the peas and cook, stirring frequently, until tender and piping hot. Stir in the pesto, yogurt and pepper, and heat through.

Drain the pasta, return to the pan and add the sauce and bacon. Toss to mix and serve sprinkled with chopped parsley or basil if you like.

Roasted sweet peppers make a delicious accompaniment. Use a mixture of red, yellow and orange peppers, quarter, core and deseed, then place in a roasting tin and brush lightly with olive oil. Roast in the oven at 190°C (375°F) Gas Mark 5 for about 45 minutes, until beginning to brown.

BONUS POINTS
• Wholemeal pasta is a better source of dietary fibre than white pasta. This helps to prevent constipation, lower blood cholesterol level and may protect against certain bowel diseases.
• Peas contain plant oestrogens that may help to balance our own level of this hormone.

OKAY FOR UNDER-ONES?
4-6 months Not suitable. See pages 16-19 for other first food ideas.
6-12 months Omit the bacon and pesto (unless you make own, see tip box). Blend the pasta with a little of the sauce (or milk if preferred). Once your baby can chew cut the pasta up small, rather than blend it.

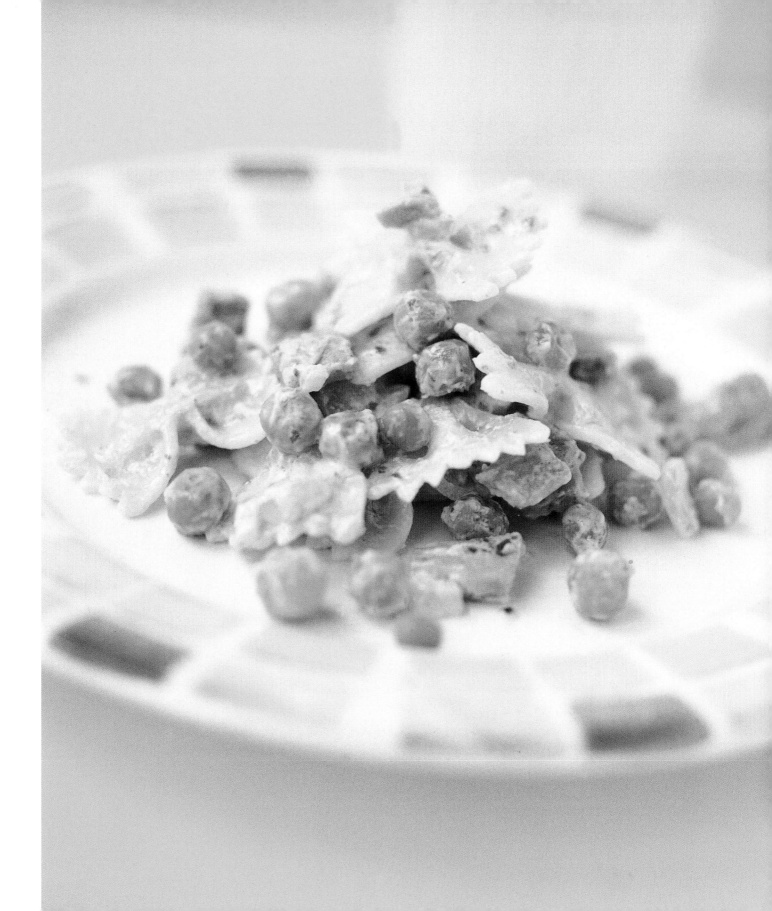

SUMMER PASTA

Children will feast their eyes on this instant and colourful pasta sauce – featuring vivid green fresh peas and courgettes, pretty pink prawns, and delicate yellow baby corn. Summer Pasta is a meal in itself, but you could serve it with a side dish of chopped tomato if you like.

250 g (8 oz) pasta shells

125 g (4 oz) baby corn, halved diagonally

150 g (5 oz) fresh shelled peas

2 tablespoons olive oil

200 g (7 oz) baby courgettes, thickly sliced

125 g (4 oz) mascarpone cheese

150 g (5 oz) shelled prawns, thawed if frozen

2-4 tablespoons chopped fresh chives (optional)

• If your children aren't keen on prawns, substitute diced ham.
• Chives may not be to everyone's taste, but you can sprinkle them over individual portions if preferred, rather than toss them with the pasta and sauce.

Cook the pasta in a large pan of boiling water for about 10 minutes until al dente – tender but firm to the bite.

Meanwhile steam the baby corn and peas in a metal steamer over boiling water for 5 minutes.

Heat the oil in a large frying pan or sauté pan. Add the courgettes and fry gently for about 3 minutes until lightly browned. Add the mascarpone and stir until melted. Add the prawns and heat through.

Lightly drain the pasta and return to the pan. Add the sauce, steamed vegetables and chives (if using) and toss together for 1 minute until heated through. Serve immediately.

BONUS POINTS
• Both pasta and peas are great for providing long-lasting energy that doesn't slump.
• The prawns, peas and cheese are all rich in calcium, which is needed for strong bones and teeth, and healthy nerves.

OKAY FOR UNDER-ONES?
4-6 months Not suitable. Instead, give a little purée made from lightly steamed courgette, perhaps with a few peas if your baby has progressed to more than one taste at a time.

6-12 months Purée the food until your baby can chew. Cooked baby corn and prawns are relatively firm, so your baby may be 10 months or so before they can manage this pasta dish cut up very small.

Note Prawns are one of the more common triggers of food allergy. If your baby hasn't tried them before, make sure they are the only new food in the dish. Then watch for unexpected symptoms (such as a rash) over the next 24-48 hours; if there are any, report them to your doctor.

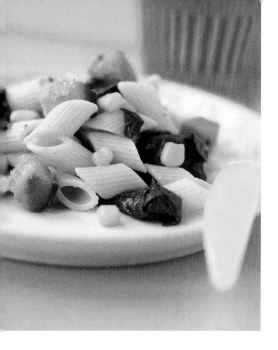

AUTUMN PASTA

Butternut squash gives this recipe its harvest-gold colour and, as the name suggests, it tastes both buttery and nutty. The peel of a ripe butternut squash is surprisingly hard, so take care that you do not cut yourself as you remove it. You will find it easier to peel if you quarter it lengthwise first.

375-425 g (12-14 oz) pasta shapes

25 g (1 oz) butter

2 tablespoons rapeseed (canola), olive or walnut oil

500 g (1 lb) butternut squash, peeled, deseeded and cut into 1 cm (½ inch) cubes

300 g (10 oz) spinach, washed and roughly torn

2 tablespoons torn fresh sage leaves

1 teaspoon freshly grated nutmeg

200 g (7 oz) can sweetcorn (preferably without salt or sugar), drained

salt (optional) and black pepper

Cook the pasta in a large pan of boiling water for about 10 minutes until al dente – tender but firm to the bite.

Meanwhile, prepare the sauce. Melt the butter with the oil in a large frying pan, add the squash and cook for about 6 minutes until softened and slightly browned.

Add the spinach, sage, nutmeg, a little salt (if using) and pepper. Cook, stirring, for a further 3 minutes. Add the sweetcorn and heat through.

Drain the pasta and add to the pan. Toss well with the sauce and serve.

BONUS POINTS
• Orange-yellow squash, such as butternut, are rich in the plant pigment beta-carotene, a valuable antioxidant that the body uses to make vitamin A. Spinach is also rich in beta-carotene.
• Sage is a veritable powerhouse of nutrients, including thujone, an antiseptic plant hormone that helps prevent infection.

OKAY FOR UNDER-ONES?
4-6 months Not suitable. Instead, give some puréed, lightly steamed butternut squash, mixed with a little milk, vegetable stock, or water.
6-12 months Omit the salt. If you can't find sweetcorn canned without salt and sugar, use cooked frozen sweetcorn instead. Blend the pasta with a little sauce. Once your baby can chew, cut the pasta up small.

• If you can't get a butternut squash, use a gem or any other edible squash; even pumpkin will do, though it's rather too watery when cooked to be a truly comparable substitute.

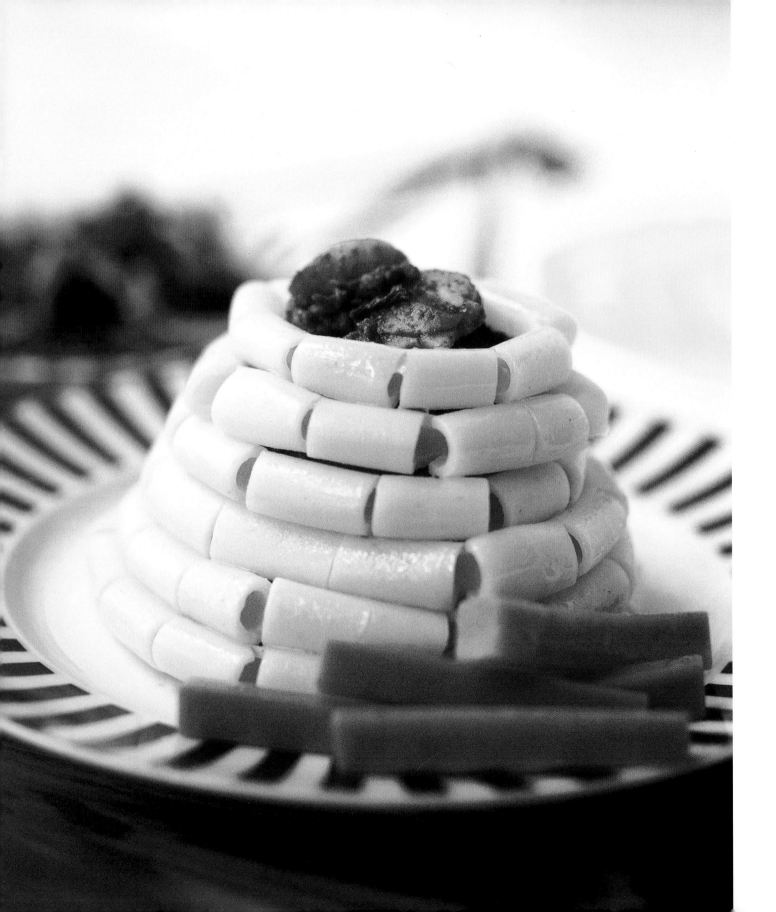

MACARONI MOUNTAIN

Making a 'mountain' by surrounding a mound of fragrant minced beef with coiled macaroni or tagliatelle presents a familiar mix of nourishing foods in a novel way to tempt children. Macaroni is popular with young children, and good for soaking up the flavour of the underlying meat and mushrooms.

1 tablespoon sunflower, rapeseed or olive oil (plus a little more for the pasta)

1 onion, chopped

1 celery stick, finely chopped

375 g (12 oz) lean minced beef

2 teaspoons tomato purée

1 tablespoon chopped fresh mixed herbs, or 1 teaspoon dried

pinch of grated nutmeg

150 ml (¼ pint) homemade vegetable stock (see page 51) or water (approximately)

375 g (12 oz) mushrooms, chopped

250 g (8 oz) bucatini (long macaroni), or tagliatelle

black pepper

Heat the oil in a large frying pan, add the onion and celery and cook gently for about 10 minutes until soft. Add the minced beef and cook, stirring, until lightly coloured. Stir in the tomato purée, herbs, nutmeg, stock and a little pepper. Cover and cook gently, stirring occasionally, for about 20-25 minutes; adding a little more stock or water during cooking if the mixture is too dry. Stir in the mushrooms and cook for a further 5 minutes or until tender.

Meanwhile, cook the pasta in a large pan of boiling water with a few drops of oil added to prevent sticking. Cook tagliatelle until al dente – tender but firm to the bite; cook macaroni until softer (to make it more flexible for shaping). Drain the cooked pasta thoroughly.

If using macaroni, spoon some mince on to each plate and form into as smooth a mound as possible. Now coil a length of cooked macaroni around the base of the mound. To keep it in place, make snips at 1 cm (½ inch) intervals around the outside, almost right across the width of the tube. Continue to coil the macaroni around the mound in a spiral fashion until you reach the top.

If using tagliatelle, simply arrange a nest of the pasta on each plate and fill with mince. Serve at once.

Steamed or boiled carrot sticks, lightly cooked shredded green cabbage and homemade tomato ketchup (see page 36) are suitable accompaniments.

BONUS POINTS
• Provides a good balance of nutrients in an attractive and unusual format.
• Pasta is good for active children because its slowly absorbed carbohydrate provides a long-lasting source of energy and steadies the blood-sugar level.

OKAY FOR UNDER-ONES?
4-6 months Not suitable. Instead, give some cooked carrot, puréed and mixed with a little milk.
Older babies Blend with a little milk or water or, once your baby can chew, cut it up small. Don't serve with tomato ketchup, unless it's homemade.

• Pasta makes this dish comfortingly familiar, but you can ring the changes. Substitute minced chicken for the beef, or create the 'mound' from a tasty mixture of Every Flavour Beans (see page 69), cooked sweetcorn kernels and steamed broccoli florets.

WINTER PASTA

If you've never thought of marrying pasta with root vegetables, you're in for a big surprise with this lovely, warming winter recipe. The sweet flavour of the parsnips and swede is further enhanced with a little chopped bacon, a ghosting of garlic and a good handful of parsley. Just try it and wait for the silence as everyone gets down to the serious business of eating.

375 g (12 oz) celeriac, pumpkin or
    squash
250 g (8 oz) small parsnips
300 g (10 oz) swede, or small turnips
2 tablespoons olive oil
1 onion, finely chopped
3 thin rashers of lean bacon, derinded
    and chopped
1 garlic clove, crushed
425 g (14 oz) can chopped tomatoes
150 ml (¼ pint) homemade chicken
    stock (see page 84) or vegetable
    stock (see page 51)
1 tablespoon clear honey (optional)
3 tablespoons chopped fresh flat leaf
    parsley (optional)
200 g (7 oz) pasta shapes
grated Cheddar cheese, to serve

• If your family enjoy their food garlicky, increase the quantity to 2 or 3 cloves.

Peel and dice the celeriac, parsnips and swede or turnips; if using pumpkin or squash, cut into wedges, deseed, cut away the skin and dice the flesh.

Heat the oil in a saucepan, add the onion and bacon and fry for about 3 minutes until lightly coloured. Add the garlic, chopped tomatoes, stock, honey (if using), vegetables and parsley. Bring to the boil, reduce the heat, cover and simmer gently for about 15 minutes or until the vegetables are tender.

Meanwhile, cook the pasta in a large pan of boiling water for about 10 minutes until al dente – tender but firm to the bite.

Drain the pasta and add to the sauce. Toss together until well combined. Serve sprinkled with cheese, and accompanied by steamed spinach, broccoli or Brussels sprout tops.

BONUS POINTS
• An easy way of giving each person two helpings of starchy carbohydrates.
• A good low-protein, high-carbohydrate meal to serve for supper – to encourage a good night's sleep.

OKAY FOR UNDER-ONES?
4-6 months Not suitable. Give a purée of one or more of the root vegetables instead.
6-12 months Choose tomatoes canned in tomato juice and without salt. Omit the honey and bacon. Purée the pasta plus sauce or, once your baby can chew, cut the food up small.

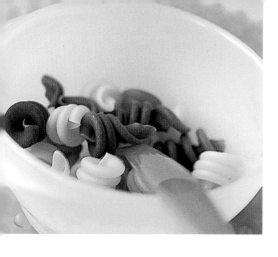

TUNA & PASTA GRATIN

Nearly everyone loves this hearty, pasta fish dish. For a change, or if you simply need a vegetarian option, try it with tofu (soy bean curd) instead of tuna. Both tuna and tofu are highly nutritious and remarkably popular with children of all ages.

250 g (8 oz) pasta shells

2 tablespoons olive oil

1 small onion, finely chopped

2 red peppers, cored, deseeded and
   diced

1 garlic clove, crushed

150 g (5 oz) cherry tomatoes, halved

15 g (½ oz) butter

50 g (2 oz) fresh wholemeal
   breadcrumbs

425 g (14 oz) can tuna in water or oil,
   drained and flaked

125 g (4 oz) mozzarella or gruyère
   cheese, grated

Cook the pasta in a large pan of boiling water for about 10 minutes until al dente – tender but firm to the bite.

Meanwhile, heat the oil in a large frying pan. Add the onion and fry gently for 3 minutes. Add the peppers and garlic and fry gently, stirring frequently, for 5 minutes. Stir in the cherry tomatoes and cook for 1 minute until softened.

Melt the butter in another pan, add the breadcrumbs and stir until evenly coated.

Drain the pasta and return to the pan. Add the pepper and tomato mixture, and the tuna. Toss together lightly, then transfer to a gratin dish.

Sprinkle with the cheese, top with the breadcrumbs and place under a preheated moderate grill for about 3-5 minutes until the cheese has melted and the breadcrumbs are golden.

Serve accompanied by steamed broccoli or green beans, and carrots.

BONUS POINTS

• Tuna contains certain omega-3 fats that help to provide the good balance of fats needed for healthy skin, blood, nerves and hormone levels. This is especially important for growing children.

• The alternative – tofu – offers a good source of vegetable protein in a soft, easy-to-eat form.

OKAY FOR UNDER-ONES?

4-6 months Not suitable. Offer some lightly steamed broccoli, green beans or carrots instead.

6-12 months Purée the pasta plus sauce, or once your baby can chew, cut it all up small. Be sure to choose tuna canned in oil or water, not in brine.

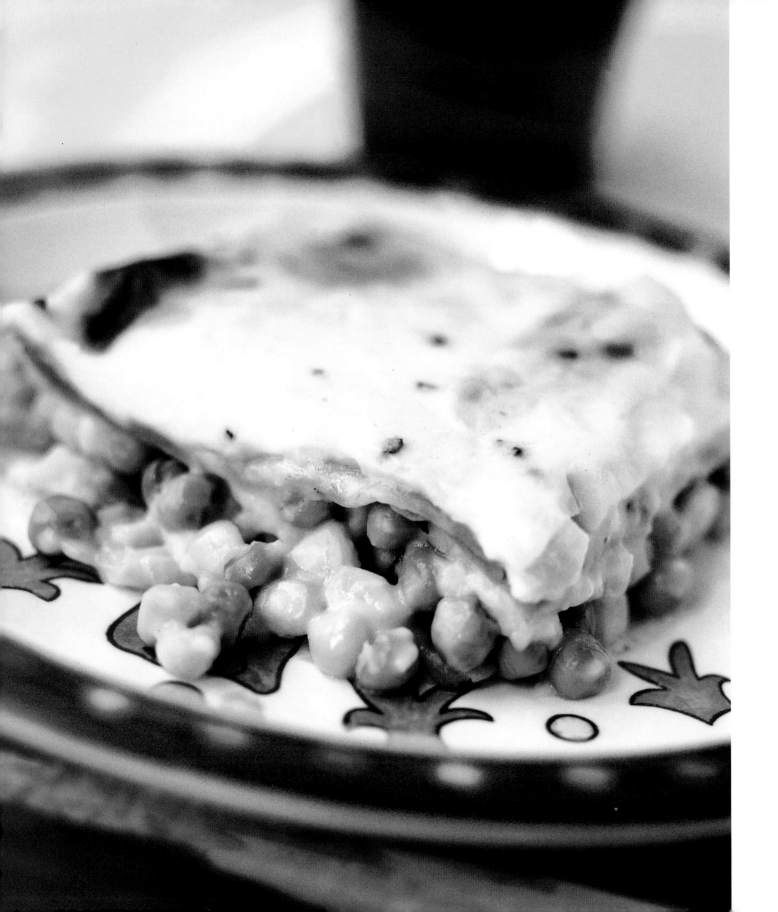

EASY PEASY LASAGNE

Green peas contrast well with golden sweetcorn to create a colourful dish that is popular with young children. Make the sauce with vegetable rather than chicken stock and you have a meal suitable for vegetarians.

50 g (2 oz) butter

2 onions, chopped

2 garlic cloves, crushed

50 g (2 oz) plain flour

600 ml (1 pint) homemade vegetable stock (see below), or chicken stock (see page 84)

300 ml (½ pint) milk

375 g (12 oz) shelled fresh or frozen green peas

250 g (8 oz) can sweetcorn (preferably without salt or sugar), drained

1 tablespoon chopped fresh parsley or mint

150 g (5 oz) ready-to-cook lasagne verdi sheets

black pepper

Melt the butter in a pan, add the onions and cook gently until soft. Add the garlic and fry for a few minutes. Stir in the flour and cook for about 1 minute. Slowly pour in the stock and milk, stirring all the time. Bring the sauce slowly to the boil, stirring constantly until thickened and smooth. Season with pepper.

If using fresh peas, par-cook in boiling water for 4-5 minutes; drain. Combine the peas and sweetcorn in a bowl and stir in the parsley or mint.

Pour a third of the sauce into a shallow ovenproof dish, then cover with a layer of lasagne sheets. Spoon the pea and sweetcorn mixture over the lasagne, then cover with half of the remaining sauce. Lay the remaining lasagne sheets on top and pour on the remaining sauce.

Bake in a preheated oven at 190°C (375°F) Gas Mark 5 for about 25 minutes until the top is golden brown and bubbling.

Serve with grilled tomatoes, steamed spinach or a green salad.

BONUS POINT
• The slow-release carbohydrate in pasta prevents tiredness and irritability from a low blood-sugar level.

OKAY FOR UNDER-ONES?
4-6 months Not suitable. See pages 16-19 for ideas for first foods.
6-12 months Use salt-free stock and full-fat milk. Blend with a little milk or water if necessary. Once your baby can chew, cut it up small. If beans and onions make your baby windy, serve for lunch rather than supper.

Vegetable stock
To make vegetable stock, put 1 small onion, chopped; 1 small carrot, chopped; ½ celery stick, finely chopped; a pinch of chopped fresh thyme or parsley; a little pepper; and 900 ml (1½ pints) water in a saucepan. Bring to the boil and simmer until the vegetables are soft, then blend until smooth.

Alternatively, you can use the (unsalted) water remaining after boiling or steaming vegetables such as spinach, carrots, cabbage or onions as stock.

Freeze stock in an ice-cube tray so you always have some nutritious liquid to moisten a baby's food. Or freeze a larger quantity in a rigid container.

PERFECT PIZZA

Pizza bases:

250 g (8 oz) strong plain white flour

250 g (8 oz) strong plain wholemeal flour

1 teaspoon caster sugar

1 sachet easy-blend active dried yeast

2 tablespoons olive oil

3 tablespoons milk

175 ml (6 fl oz) hand-hot water
    (approximately)

Tomato and garlic topping:

2 tablespoons olive or corn oil

2 garlic cloves, crushed

500 g (1 lb) tomatoes, skinned if
    preferred, chopped

4 tablespoons tomato paste, preferably
    sun-dried (optional)

2 tablespoons chopped fresh oregano,
    or 2 teaspoons dried

12 pitted black olives (optional)

300 g (10 oz) mozzarella cheese, finely
    sliced

black pepper

2 tablespoons extra-virgin olive oil for
    sprinkling (optional)

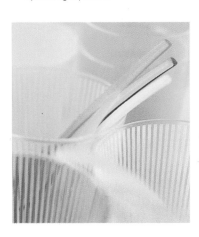

Homemade pizzas are much more delicious than shop-bought ones and they are easy to make. You need to allow at least 1 hour for the dough to rise. This topping is very simple; for more elaborate toppings, *see page 54.*

To make the pizza dough, put the flours in a large bowl and stir in the sugar and yeast. Make a well in the centre and add the oil, milk and water. Mix to a smooth, pliable dough that forms a ball and leaves the sides of the bowl clean. If the dough is too floury, add a little more milk; if it's too wet, add a little more flour. Knead for 5 minutes, then place in a clean bowl, cover with a tea towel and leave to rise in a warm place (such as an airing cupboard) for 1 hour. (At room temperature, the dough may take about 2 hours to rise.)

Knead the risen dough a little to 'knock back' (release air), then break into 4 pieces. Press each into a thin round; carefully transfer to oiled baking sheets.

To make the topping, heat the oil in a large frying pan, add the garlic and fry gently for 1 minute. Add the tomatoes and fry for 3-4 minutes, stirring frequently. Season with pepper.

Prick the pizza bases all over with a fork, then spread a tablespoon of tomato paste evenly on each one. Divide the garlic and tomato mixture between the bases, spreading it to the edges. Leave the pizzas to stand for a further 20 minutes so they rise a little.

Bake the pizzas in the preheated oven at 200°C (400°F) Gas Mark 6 for 15 minutes. Sprinkle with oregano and the olives (if using). Lay the mozzarella slices on top. Sprinkle with olive oil if required. Bake for a further 10 minutes until the cheese is melted and bubbling. Accompany with a salad if you like.

BONUS POINTS
• Using some wholemeal flour in pizza bases increases your family's fibre intake, which among other things is good for digestion.
• The popular combination of tomatoes and onions provides valuable nutrients that offer some protection from coughs, colds and other infections.

OKAY FOR UNDER-ONES?
Don't use tomato paste or olives.
4-6 months Not suitable. See pages 16-19 for ideas for first foods.
6-9 months Blend some pizza with a little milk or water, or, for babies who can chew, cut up small and soften with a little milk or water.
9-12 months Older babies can usually hold a piece of pizza in their hands.

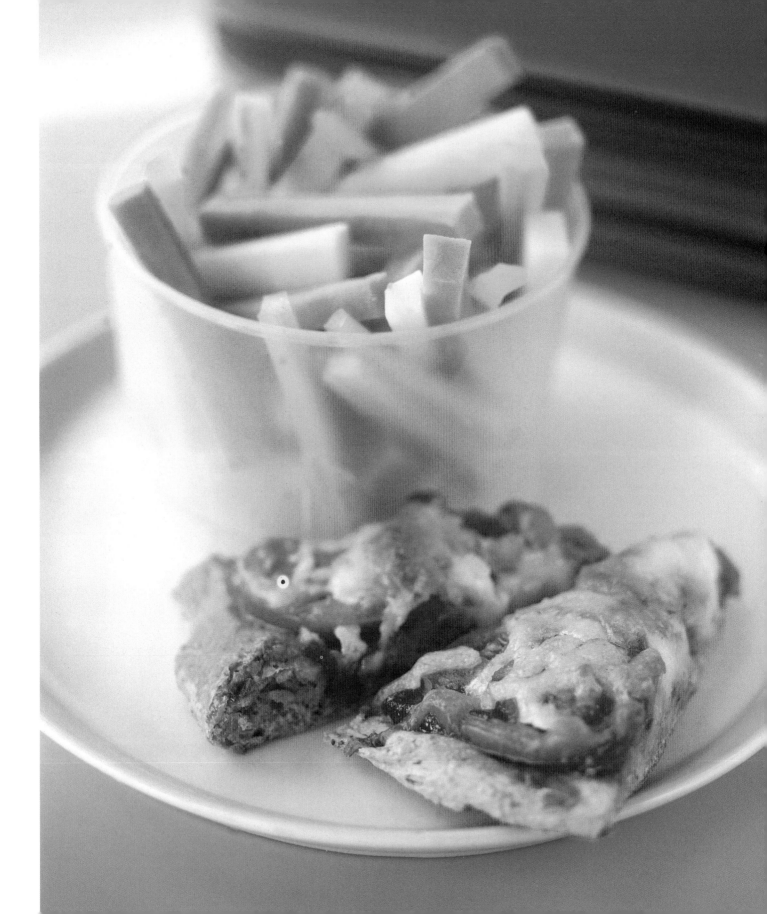

CHICKEN, SWEETCORN & PINEAPPLE PIZZA

4 basic pizza bases (see page 52)

250 g (8 oz) frozen sweetcorn kernels

4 tablespoons olive oil

2 onions, finely chopped

2 boneless, skinless chicken breasts,
    thinly sliced

1 teaspoon medium curry paste
    (optional)

75 g (3 oz) cream cheese

4 slices of fresh pineapple, peeled, cored
    and chopped

75 g (3 oz) Cheddar cheese, grated

Add the sweetcorn to a pan of boiling water, bring back to the boil and simmer for 2 minutes; drain.

Heat the oil in a large frying pan. Add the onions and fry gently for 3-4 minutes until golden. Add the chicken and fry gently for 5 minutes or until it is cooked through. Stir in the curry paste (if using) and sweetcorn.

Dot the cream cheese over the pizza bases to within 1 cm (½ inch) of the edges. Spread with the chicken and sweetcorn mixture. Scatter with the chopped pineapple, then the grated Cheddar. Leave to rise for 20 minutes.

Bake in a preheated oven at 200°C (400°F) Gas Mark 6 for 20 minutes until the topping is golden.

BONUS POINTS

• A nutritious pizza topping that provides plenty of protein and vitamins.

OKAY FOR UNDER-ONES?

4-6 months Not suitable. Instead give a little puréed pineapple, or sweetcorn. Babies of 5 months and older could have some puréed chicken.

6-9 months Blend some pizza with a little milk or water, or, for babies who can chew, cut up small and soften with a little milk or water.

9-12 months Older babies can usually hold a piece of pizza in their hands.

ROASTED VEGETABLE PIZZA

4 basic pizza bases (see page 52)

4 medium courgettes

2 red or orange peppers, cored,
    deseeded and sliced

2 red onions, finely chopped

4 tablespoons olive oil

125 g (4 oz) button mushrooms,
    thinly sliced

200 g (7 oz) cherry tomatoes, halved

250 g (8 oz) mozzarella cheese,
    thinly sliced

75 g (3 oz) Cheddar cheese, grated

Slice the courgettes diagonally and scatter in a roasting tin with the peppers and red onions. Drizzle with the oil and bake in a preheated oven at 220°C (425°F) Gas Mark 7 for 25 minutes or until lightly coloured. Add the mushrooms and cherry tomatoes, stir and roast for a further 10 minutes.

Scatter the mozzarella cheese and roasted vegetables over the pizza bases to within 1 cm (½ inch) of the edges. Sprinkle the grated Cheddar on top and leave to rise for 20 minutes. Bake for 15-20 minutes until golden.

BONUS POINTS

• Red peppers and tomatoes are a valuable source of vitamin C and beta-carotene, while mushrooms supply vitamin B.

OKAY FOR UNDER-ONES?

4-6 months Not suitable. Give some puréed courgettes instead.

6-9 months Blend some pizza with a little milk or water, or, for babies who can chew, cut up small and soften with a little milk or water.

9-12 months Older babies can usually hold a piece of pizza in their hands.

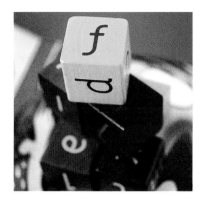

FRENCH BREAD PIZZAS

These pizzas are a quick and easy standby for lunch during a busy weekend, and most people eat them with their hands, which cuts down on washing up! All you need is a French stick (baguette) and pizza topping – either the speedy cheese and tomato topping below, or one of those suggested for the traditional pizzas on pages 52-54. It doesn't matter if the bread is a day old, for the topping soon sinks in and transforms it into a fragrant repast.

15-20 cm (6-8 inch) piece French stick per person

Topping:
3 tablespoons tomato ketchup, preferably homemade (see page 36)
375 g (12 oz) tomatoes, sliced
200 g (7 oz) mozzarella cheese, thinly sliced
12 pitted black olives (optional)

Split the lengths of French stick in half lengthways and lay, cut side up, in a roasting tin. Spread evenly with the tomato ketchup, then cover with the sliced tomatoes and mozzarella. Add the olives (if using). Rest the pizzas against each other so their upper surfaces are as flat as possible; this helps to keep the topping from slipping off as the pizzas are cooking.

Bake in a preheated oven at 180°C (350°F) Gas Mark 4 for 15 minutes until the cheese is melted and bubbling. Serve warm, with a crisp lettuce salad if you like.

BONUS POINTS
• French bread is an excellent vehicle for a nutritious topping. Tomatoes, for example, are a valuable source of beta-carotene and vitamin C.

OKAY FOR UNDER-ONES?
Don't use bought tomato ketchup or olives.
4-6 months Not suitable. See pages 16-19 for ideas for first foods.
6-9 months Blend with a little milk or water or, for babies who can chew, cut up small and soften with a little milk or water.
9-12 months Older babies can usually hold a small piece of French Bread pizza in their hands. The bread at the base can be rather hard, but a baby will eat the soft bits first, then deal with the remaining hard bread as if it were a rusk, by sucking on it until it is soft enough to eat.

• A white baguette is fine, but a wholemeal baguette – available from selected supermarkets and bakers – provides more fibre, 'bite' and taste
• It's better to cook these pizzas in a roasting tin than on a baking tray, as the support from the sides of the tin helps keep them steady.

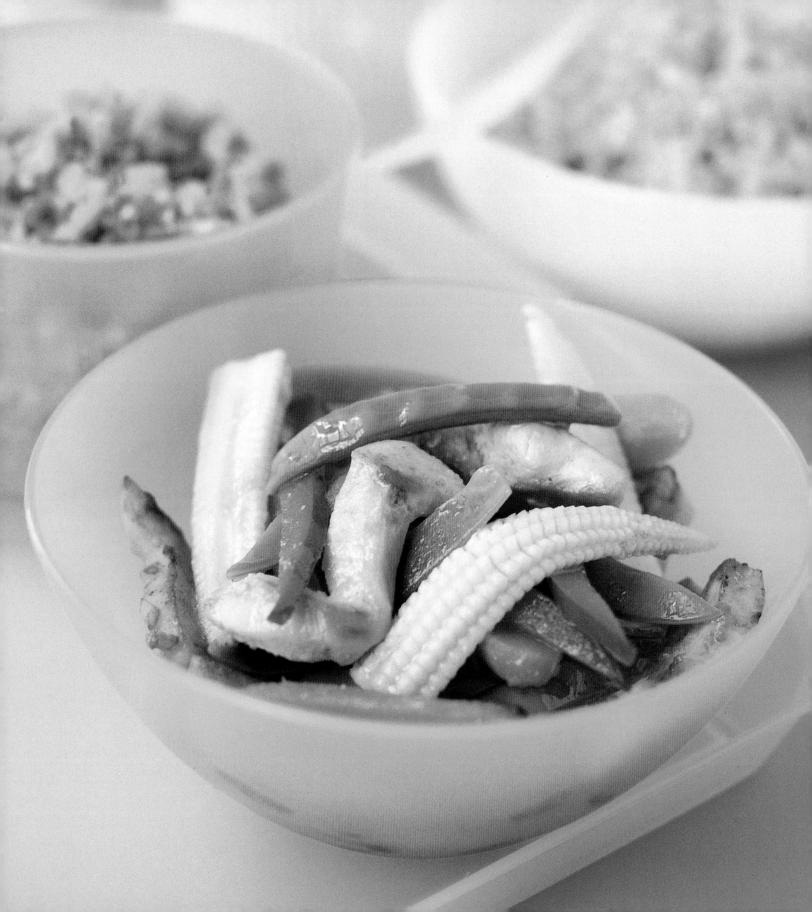

Good Food Fast

There are occasions when you have plenty of time to cook, but more often than not you need a meal on the table as quickly as possible. This is one way you can find time to share your children's activities, or just relax and restore your energy. These recipes are simple, appealing and nutritious.

BABY VEGETABLE & CHICKEN STIR-FRY

Stir-frying makes vegetables taste more attractive – even to the most reluctant child – because it brings out their natural sweetness.

500 g (1 lb) skinless, boneless chicken breast

175 g (6 oz) baby carrots, scraped

175 g (6 oz) baby corn, halved lengthways

3 tablespoons sunflower oil

1 red pepper, cored, deseeded and thinly sliced lengthways

1 garlic clove, crushed

175 g (6 oz) small mangetout

Cut the chicken into thin strips across the grain; set aside. Blanch the carrots in boiling water for 2 minutes. Lift out with a slotted spoon, immediately refresh under cold running water, then drain. Repeat with the baby corn.

Heat 2 tablespoons of the oil in a wok or large, deep frying pan over a moderate heat. Add the chicken strips, increase the heat to high and stir-fry for 3-4 minutes or until lightly coloured on all sides. Remove the chicken with a slotted spoon and transfer to a plate.

Heat the remaining oil in the wok on a moderate heat. Add the red pepper and garlic and stir-fry for 2-3 minutes until softened, but not coloured.

Add the carrots, corn and mangetout. Increase heat to high and stir-fry for 3-4 minutes, until tinged brown. Add the chicken and its juices and toss over the heat for 1 minute. Serve with rice, preferably nutty brown rice.

BONUS POINTS
• Provides one of the 5 recommended daily helpings of vegetables and fruit.
• A valuable source of fibre – to keep the bowel in good working order.

OKAY FOR UNDER-ONES?
4-6 months Not suitable. Give some mashed cooked carrots, moistened with a little homemade vegetable stock (see page 51) or chicken stock (see page 84).
6-12 months Blend or mince the stir-fry until your baby is able to chew small pieces of chicken, baby corn and mangetout – probably around 10 months, then cut the food up small.

• For over-ones, you can enhance the flavour of this stir-fry by adding up to 4 tablespoons of yellow bean sauce and 1 tablespoon of sherry vinegar before returning the chicken to the wok.

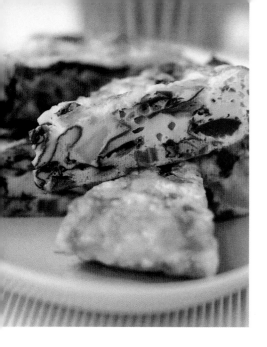

FRITTATA

A quick-cooking Italian frittata is rather like a Spanish omelette – and you can make it more so by adding chunks of cooked potato if you like. It is an ideal choice when you need a hearty meal in minutes and, as an added bonus, most young children love it. You will need a frying pan that is suitable for use under the grill.

If including potato, cook in lightly salted boiling water for 6-8 minutes or until just tender. Drain thoroughly.

Melt the butter with the oil in a large non-stick frying pan. Add the onion, celery and red pepper and fry for 5-6 minutes, until soft and slightly browned. Add the spinach and cook for a further 2-3 minutes, until wilted. Stir in the potato if using.

Season the beaten eggs with pepper, then pour over the vegetables in the pan. Cook over a medium heat for about 5 minutes until the base is set.

Sprinkle the cheese on top of the frittata. Place under a preheated grill for 2-3 minutes until the cheese is melted and the top is set and golden brown.

Serve hot or warm, with crusty bread and a cucumber or tomato salad.

BONUS POINTS

• Eggs are a good source of complete protein, so this is a valuable dish for vegetarians.
• Spinach is rich in plant pigments such as beta-carotene, chlorophyll, lutein and xanthine (good for immunity, eyes and skin); and minerals, notably calcium and magnesium; it is also a useful source of iron.

OKAY FOR UNDER-ONES?

4-6 months Not suitable. Instead, give some boiled potato, mashed with a little milk, vegetable water, or water.
6-12 months Use only 1 stick of celery, and half the amount of spinach. Blend the frittata with a little milk, vegetable water, or water. Or, once your baby can chew, simply cut it up into small pieces.

175 g (6 oz) potato, cut into 2.5 cm
    (1 inch) chunks (optional)
25 g (1 oz) butter
1 tablespoon olive, rapeseed (canola) or
    walnut oil
1 onion, (preferably red), finely sliced
2 celery sticks, chopped
1 red pepper, halved, cored, deseeded
    and chopped
250 g (8 oz) baby spinach, trimmed and
    washed
6 eggs, beaten
75 g (3 oz) Cheddar cheese, grated
salt (optional) and black pepper

• If preferred, substitute lightly steamed chopped broccoli florets for spinach.

BUBBLE & SQUEAK

Bubble and squeak is an old family favourite and easy to prepare. It takes its name from the bubbling of the butter followed by the 'squeaking' of the cooked greens and potatoes as they're fried until golden brown and crispy at the edges.

50 g (2 oz) butter

1 tablespoon olive oil

500 g (1 lb) boiled potato, cut into chunks or roughly mashed

500 g (1 lb) cooked cabbage, spring greens or Brussels sprouts

salt (optional) and black pepper

Melt the butter with the oil in a large non-stick frying pan. Add the potato and cabbage, spring greens or Brussels sprouts. Season with a little salt (if using) and pepper.

Fry, stirring occasionally with a wooden spoon, until golden brown underneath and crispy at the edges. Serve on its own, or with ham or other cold meat.

BONUS POINTS

• Cabbage, spring greens and Brussels sprouts contain many valuable nutrients, including vitamin C and calcium.

OKAY FOR UNDER-ONES?

It's normal for babies to have some wind after eating greens. To avoid the risk of an interrupted night's sleep, make this recipe for your baby's lunch rather than supper.

4-6 months Not suitable. Give some mashed boiled potato, moistened with a little milk or water.

6-12 months Do not add salt. Blend the food with a little milk or water or, once your baby can chew, cut into pieces. Serve with cold chicken rather than ham (blended or cut up).

• For older children and adults add a spicy note, by frying 1 teaspoon of crushed coriander seeds in the butter and oil for 1 minute before adding the vegetables.

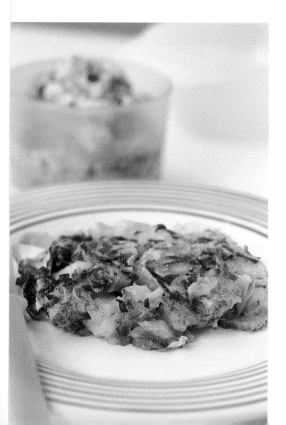

HOT CATS

Fast foods, such as burgers and hot dogs, are perennial favourites and easy for everyone to eat with their fingers. Creating your own fun versions is guaranteed to delight young children.

4 pieces of fresh skinless cod, each 75 g
    (3 oz), or frozen fish steaks, thawed
4 long, soft rolls or 8 bridge rolls, or
    4 baps
2 tablespoons mayonnaise
2 tablespoons Greek yogurt
handful of Romaine or Cos lettuce leaves
1 large or 2 small gherkins, sliced
    (optional)

Steam the fish in a steamer over a pan of simmering water or poach in a shallow pan containing a 1cm (½ inch) depth of simmering water for 8-10 minutes until just tender.

Split open the rolls or baps, but do not cut right through. Mix the mayonnaise and yogurt together in a small bowl, then spread on the cut surfaces of each roll or bap. Lay 1 or 2 lettuce leaves on each bottom half, add a few gherkin slices (if using), then insert the fish fillets, cutting to fit as necessary. Serve with green beans or peas, oven-baked chips and tomato ketchup, preferably homemade (see page 36).

BONUS POINTS
• From a nutritional angle, 'hot cats' are rich in protein (essential for growth and cell repair) and vitamin B (good for nerve function).

OKAY FOR UNDER-ONES?
Check fish carefully for bones, even though it is sold as filleted.
4-6 months Not suitable. See pages 16-19 for other ideas.
6-12 months Blend with a little milk or water or, once your baby can chew, cut up small and moisten if necessary with a little milk or water.

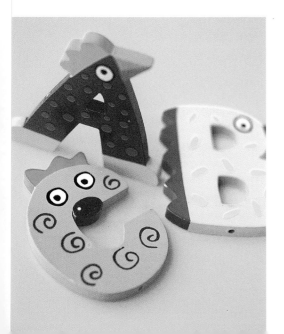

• Choose wholemeal bread for its superior flavour and higher fibre content.
• Use low-fat mayonnaise for those who are reducing their fat intake.
• Grill or bake the fish if preferred, but steaming or poaching keeps it moist.
• For a more piquant flavour, you can replace 1 tablespoon of the mayonnaise with 1 tablespoon tartare sauce (but not for under-ones).

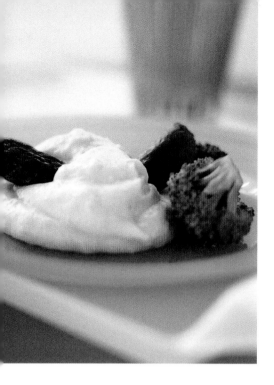

SILLY SAUSAGES

Serve ever-popular sausages in an original way to give them a little more verve and boost their child-appeal. High quality sausages – with less fat and rusk filler than the average sausage – are now widely available from good butchers and supermarkets. These have a higher percentage of lean meat and some contain other ingredients, such as leeks.

750 g (1½ lb) potatoes
a little milk
8 good-quality sausages
1-2 tablespoons corn oil
salt (optional)

To serve (optional):
tomato ketchup, preferably homemade
(see page 36)

Cook the potatoes in lightly salted (or unsalted) water until tender. Drain and mash thoroughly with a little milk.

Meanwhile, prick each sausage with a fork in 3 places. Heat the oil in a non-stick frying pan, add the sausages and fry, turning occasionally, for 10-20 minutes, depending on thickness, until cooked through.

Cut each sausage in half widthways. Make a mound of mashed potato on each plate, then stick 4 sausage halves into each mound, cut end downwards, rather like the Millennium Dome! Serve with tomato ketchup if you like. Suitable accompaniments are green beans, broccoli or peas; and Every Flavour Beans (see page 69) or canned baked beans.

BONUS POINT
• Sausages are a good source of protein and energy.

OKAY FOR UNDER-ONES?
Sausages are usually high in salt and are therefore generally unsuitable for babies.

4-6 months Not suitable. Give some boiled potato, mashed with a little milk or water.

6-12 months Only sausages without added salt are suitable and these aren't easy to obtain unless, of course, you make your own. If available, either blend cooked sausages and potato with some milk or water or, once your baby can chew, cut up small. Serve with peas or Brussels sprouts, blended or cut up, but don't give canned baked beans or ready-made tomato ketchup.

• Sausages are typically high in fat, so prune the fat content of the rest of the meal. Choose low-fat sausages if possible. Drain the sausages on kitchen paper after frying, to remove excess fat, or grill them instead.

POPEYE'S PORK

500 g (1 lb) small red 'salad' potatoes, scrubbed

500 g (1 lb) pork escalopes

2 tablespoons olive oil

1 red onion, chopped

1 garlic clove, crushed

150 ml (¼ pint) homemade vegetable stock (see page 51) or chicken stock (see page 84)

175 g (6 oz) fromage frais

200 g (7 oz) baby spinach, trimmed and washed

Many people believe spinach is the best source of iron, but this isn't the case. A higher level of iron was mistakenly assigned to spinach in a nutrient table some time ago, and this mistake was copied many times! However, spinach does contain some iron, as well as magnesium, calcium and plant pigments – all of which children need for everyday health and strength.

Halve any large potatoes to give even-sized chunks. Steam over boiling water for 15 minutes until just tender. Meanwhile, press the pork between pieces of kitchen paper to remove excess moisture, then cut into thin strips.

Heat the oil in a large sauté pan or wok. Add the pork and fry quickly until seared on all sides, about 3 minutes. Add the onion and garlic and fry, stirring, for a further 3-4 minutes until softened.

Add the stock and fromage frais. Cover and simmer gently for 5 minutes. Add the potatoes and spinach and cook gently, stirring the spinach into the cooking juices until wilted. Serve immediately.

Beetroot is a good accompaniment to this dish: simply boil raw beetroot until soft, rub off their skins, then grate to serve.

BONUS POINTS
• Pork is a good source of protein (essential for growth) and vitamin B (for healthy nerves).
• Onion and garlic are both believed to contain anti-viral and anti-bacterial agents that can help fight infection.

OKAY FOR UNDER-ONES?
4-6 months Not suitable. Give some mashed potato or puréed spinach instead or, for babies used to several tastes together, a combination of the two. Moisten the vegetables with homemade chicken or vegetable stock.
6-12 months Cut the cooked pork up small, then blend all the food together. Alternatively, for babies who can cope with lumps, mince the pork and mash the rest. Your baby will probably be around 10 months before he or she can chew little pieces of pork, however small you cut them.

> • Yellow-skinned potatoes are a good alternative to red ones. The skins of both red and yellow-skinned potatoes contain more plant pigments than do those of ordinary 'white' potatoes.

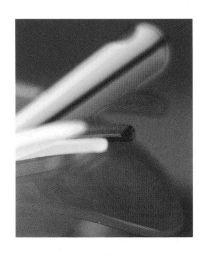

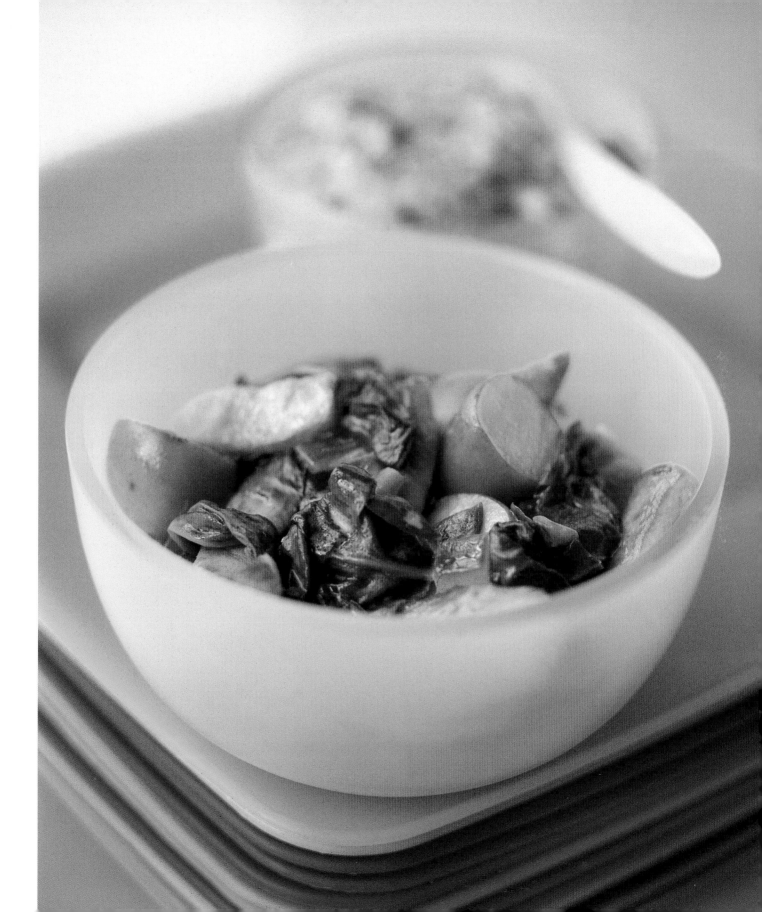

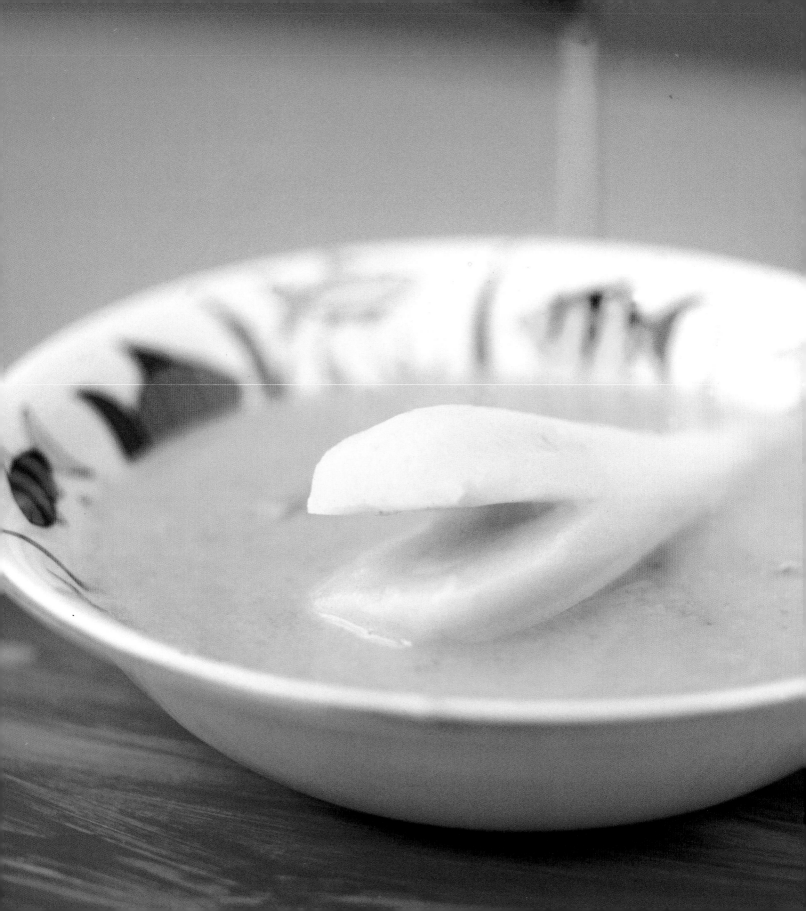

Anytime Fillers

The versatile recipes in this chapter provide for all kinds of meals, from lunches, through high teas to suppers. At times, a child simply needs something extra in their tummy between meals, especially if there are 5 or 6 hours between lunch and supper. Fruit, cereal bars and sandwiches are possibilities, but they might well require something more substantial. Here are lots of ideas to fit the bill, including Sweetcorn Griddle Cakes, Every Flavour Beans, and simple but superb milk shakes.

SHARK SOUP

4 small or medium parsnips
25 g (1 oz) butter
1 onion, chopped
1.2 litres (2 pints) fresh chicken stock
    (preferably homemade, see page 84)
500 g (1 lb) shelled fresh, or frozen peas
small pinch of freshly grated nutmeg
1 tablespoon cornflour, mixed with
    2 tablespoons water
black pepper
shredded fresh mint leaves, to garnish

Have fun with this soup by shaping parsnips to resemble sharks' jaws. Each parsnip is placed in a bowl of soup so it looks as if it's swimming in a pea-green sea. If your children aren't keen on parsnips, use carrots instead.

With a sharp knife, cut a wedge from the base of each parsnip to resemble an open jaw. Steam the parsnips or boil in water for about 20 minutes until tender.

Meanwhile, melt the butter in a large saucepan, add the onion and fry gently, stirring frequently, for about 5 minutes until softened but not browned. Add the stock, peas, nutmeg and pepper. Stir in the blended cornflour. Bring to the boil, partially cover and simmer for 10 minutes, stirring occasionally.

Let cool slightly, then purée the soup in a blender. Reheat if necessary to serve. Pour some soup into each warmed shallow soup bowl. Lay a parsnip 'shark' in each bowl and sprinkle the pea-soup 'sea' with shredded mint to resemble seaweed. Serve with wholemeal bread, and perhaps cheese.

BONUS POINTS
• Parsnips are a good source of fibre, and contain vitamins C and E.
• Plant hormones in peas may help balance some of our own hormones.

OKAY FOR UNDER-ONES?
Use chicken stock that doesn't contain salt.
4-6 months Blend some parsnip with a little milk or water; for a 5 month-old, add a teaspoon of soup to the purée as well.
6-12 months Cook the parsnip until soft; mash it into the soup. When your baby can chew, cut the parsnip up small.

• Check that the parsnips are tender with a knife before adding them to the soup; older parsnips take longer to cook.
• Use homegrown fresh peas during their short summer season – they have a far superior flavour to frozen ones.

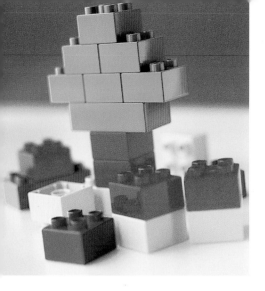

CHICKEN SOUP

Whenever you roast a chicken, don't throw away the carcass – use it to make a nourishing soup instead. Homemade chicken soup has long had a reputation for helping to fight colds and other infections. This tasty soup can also be made using a raw chicken carcass or bones (see tip box).

1 roast chicken carcass

jellied chicken stock (see tip box)

1 tablespoon vinegar

1 tablespoon chicken fat (see tip box)

2 carrots, cut into large chunks

1 parsnip, cut into large chunks

1 onion, quartered

1-2 garlic cloves

1 celery stick, finely sliced

2 tablespoons red lentils

4 tablespoons single cream

125 g (4 oz) cooked chicken breast,
    skinned and shredded (optional)

black pepper

chopped fresh parsley, to serve

• After roasting a chicken, pour the juices from the roasting pan into a bowl and allow to cool. The liquid will separate into 2 layers: a clear layer of jellied stock, with a layer of chicken fat on top.

• Instead of using a cooked chicken carcass, you can make this soup with 1.6 kg (3½ lb) raw chicken bones. Proceed as above, but simmer for a full 3 hours.

Put the chicken carcass in a large saucepan and add sufficient water to cover. Bring to the boil. Put on the lid, leaving a small gap for steam to escape, and simmer very gently for at least 1 hour, preferably 2-3 hours.

Strain the broth through a fine sieve to remove the bones, and return to the rinsed-out pan. Add the jellied stock, vinegar, chicken fat, carrots, parsnip, onion, garlic, celery, lentils and pepper, and bring back to the boil. Simmer, partially covered, for 30 minutes.

Remove from the heat and add a little water if necessary to make up the volume to about 1.2 litres (2 pints).

Use a slotted spoon to lift the vegetables and lentils from the broth and transfer to a blender. Add the cream and a little of the broth, and blend until smooth. Add the puréed vegetables to the broth in the pan and stir well. Stir in the chicken (if using).

Ladle the soup into warmed bowls and sprinkle with chopped parsley. Serve with crusty wholemeal bread.

BONUS POINTS
• Research has shown that homemade chicken soup helps clear a bunged-up nose, reduces inflammation, and improves immunity.
• The lentils used to help thicken the soup provide fibre and slow-release carbohydrate that deters hunger for several hours.

OKAY FOR UNDER-ONES?
For babies that get very windy, leave out the lentils. Take care to search for and remove any stray chicken bones. Don't serve with wholemeal bread if your baby is under 6 months.

4-6 months Remove some cooked carrot or parsnip, and blend with a little milk or liquid from the unblended soup. Babies of 5 months can have a tiny bit of chicken, blended with some carrot or parsnip, and a little of the soup liquid.

6-10 months Give the soup as it is (without added chicken meat), or blend some soup with a little chicken.

10-12 months Cut cooked chicken up small before adding to the soup.

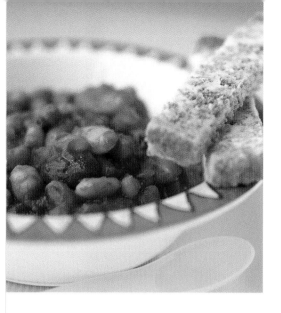

EVERY FLAVOUR BEANS

Many of us love canned baked beans, but it's really easy to cook your own at home – and, better still, you can then make them any flavour you like, including sweet, spicy and tangy.

250 g (8 oz) dried cannellini, flageolet, borlotti, black-eyed, red kidney or haricot beans, soaked overnight in cold water

2 onions, chopped

2 garlic cloves, crushed

1 tablespoon black treacle, molasses or dark muscovado sugar

4 tablespoons tomato purée (optional)

1 tablespoon Dijon mustard (optional)

1 teaspoon Worcestershire sauce (optional)

Drain the beans, rinse and place in a large saucepan. Add plenty of cold water to cover, bring to the boil and fast-boil for 10 minutes, the lower the heat and simmer for 1-2 hours until tender. Drain well.

Put the beans into a casserole and add the remaining ingredients, along with enough boiling water to just cover. Put a lid on the casserole and cook in a preheated oven at 180°C (350°F) Gas Mark 4 for 30 minutes. Remove the lid, stir gently, then cook for a further 30 minutes.

VARIATIONS

Spicy beans Add ¼-½ teaspoon of chilli powder to the beans together with the other ingredients.

Tangy beans Add 2 tablespoons of chutney and an extra 1-2 teaspoons of Worcestershire sauce to the beans together with the other ingredients.

Honeyed beans Add 2 tablespoons of clear honey to the beans together with the other ingredients.

Bacon-flavoured beans Add 250 g (8 oz) bacon, derinded and chopped, to the beans together with the other ingredients.

BONUS POINTS
• The proteins and plant hormones in beans make them valuable for growth and for helping to balance the level of our own oestrogen.
• Beans also contain slowly absorbed carbohydrate that sustains you for longer and helps steady blood-sugar level.

OKAY FOR UNDER-ONES?
4-6 months Not suitable. See pages 16-19 for other ideas.
6-12 months The basic recipe is suitable but not the variations. Blend or, once your baby can chew, cut the beans up small. It's normal for babies to be windy after eating beans, but you may find it better to serve them for lunch rather than supper to ensure night sleep isn't affected.

• For a speedy alternative, you can use a 475 g (15 oz) can beans. Put these straight into the casserole. Fry the onion in a little oil until soft before adding, and reduce the cooking time in the oven by half.
• The cooking time for pulses can vary enormously, depending on the variety and how long they have been stored.

BAKED POTATOES WITH CAULIFLOWER CHEESE

Scooped-out baked potatoes make excellent cases for various fillings – here tasty cauliflower cheese makes a perfect partner for bland potato. Baked potato skins are delicious in themselves, so encourage everyone except under-twos to enjoy their chewy texture rather than leave them on the side of their plate.

4 large baking potatoes

olive oil, for brushing

1 cauliflower, cut into florets

15 g (½ oz) butter

15 g (½ oz) plain flour

300 ml (½ pint) milk

125 g (4 oz) Cheddar cheese, grated

black pepper

• Reduce the fat content of this dish by using semi-skimmed milk if your children are all over 2 years.

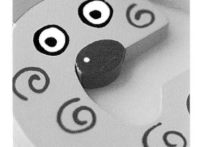

Prick the potatoes in several places, place on a baking tray, and brush all over with the oil. Bake in a preheated oven at 190°C (375°F) Gas Mark 5 for 1½ hours, until they feel soft when pressed.

Meanwhile, steam the cauliflower in a steamer over boiling water for 8 minutes.

Melt the butter in a saucepan, then stir in the flour. Cook, stirring, for 2 minutes. Whisk in the milk, a little at a time, and cook, stirring, to make a smooth thick sauce. Stir in about three quarters of the cheese and season with a little pepper. Gently stir in the cauliflower.

Cut the baked potatoes in half, and scoop out most of the potato, leaving a shell about 1cm (½ inch) thick. Return to the baking tray. Pile the cauliflower cheese mixture into the potato shells and sprinkle the remaining cheese on top. Bake for 20 minutes.

Raw carrots, sliced lengthways, are perfect for dipping into the hot cauliflower cheese filling.

BONUS POINTS
• Cheese is an excellent source of protein (for growth and repair) and calcium (for strong bones and teeth).
• Potato skins are rich in fibre, encouraging a steady level of blood sugar, and a low level of cholesterol. Fibre also helps to prevent constipation.

OKAY FOR UNDER-ONES?
4-6 months Mash some of the scooped-out cooked potato or cauliflower with a little milk or water, or offer both.
6-12 months Mash scooped-out potato with the cauliflower cheese or, for babies who can chew, cut the potato and cauliflower up small.

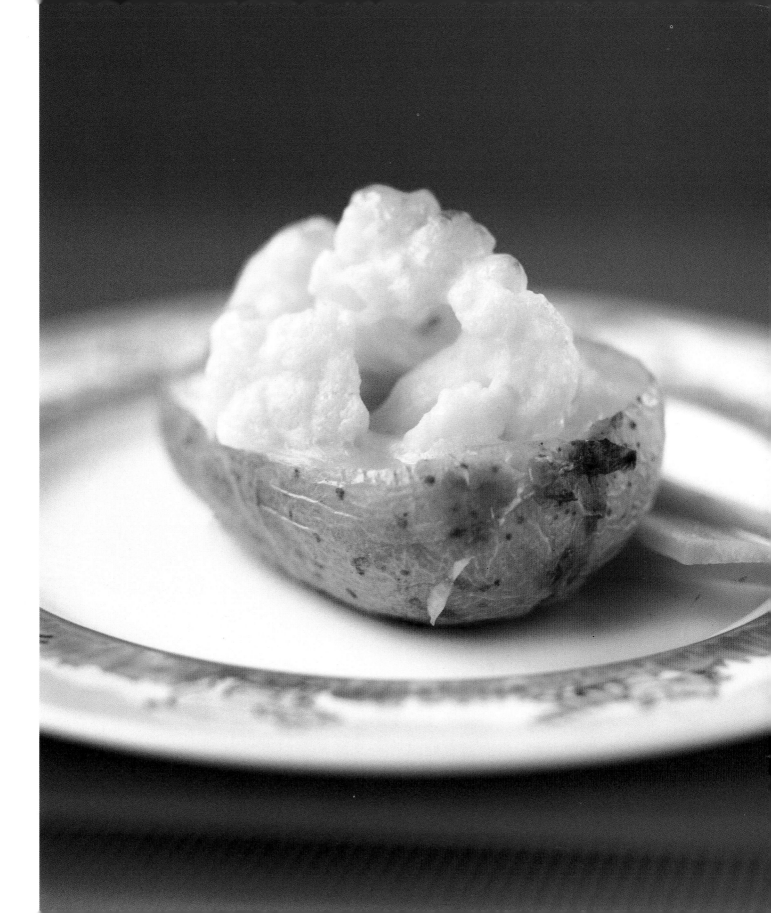

SAGE & SQUASH GNOCCHI

You'll be delighted when you taste these little Italian dumplings for the first time. Butter and fragrant sage complement the smooth squash and potato mash, to excellent effect.

375 g (12 oz) butternut squash, peeled and cubed

250 g (8 oz) potatoes, peeled and cubed

1 egg yolk

125 g (4 oz) plain flour, plus extra if required

pinch of freshly grated nutmeg

75 g (3 oz) unsalted butter

1-2 tablespoons torn fresh sage leaves (optional)

salt (optional) and black pepper

grated Gruyère or Cheddar cheese, to serve

Cook the squash and potatoes in boiling water to cover for 10-15 minutes, or until tender. Meanwhile, bring another large pan of water to the boil.

Drain the squash and potatoes thoroughly, then mash them well together. Beat in the egg yolk, flour, nutmeg, pinch of salt (if using) and black pepper to form a soft, moist gnocchi dough. Add a little extra flour if needed to obtain the required consistency.

Now drop 8-10 separate heaped teaspoonfuls of this dough into the pan of boiling water, keeping them well apart, and boil for 1-2 minutes until they rise to the surface. Lift out with a slotted spoon, and place in a warmed bowl; keep warm while cooking the rest of the mixture in batches in the same way.

Melt the butter in a large frying pan, add the sage (if using) and cook for 1 minute. Add the gnocchi, toss carefully to coat them with the butter, and heat through.

Serve the gnocchi sprinkled with grated cheese. Accompany with fresh tomato sauce, or homemade pesto (see page 42) if you like.

BONUS POINTS
• Squash is rich in beta-carotene, the vitamin-A precursor that is an excellent antioxidant and especially beneficial to the skin and lining of the lungs.

OKAY FOR UNDER-ONES?
Omit the salt.
4-6 months Not suitable. Instead, steam some squash or potato and mash or blend with a little milk or water.
6-12 months Blend the gnocchi with a little milk or water. Or, once your baby can chew, cut them up small.

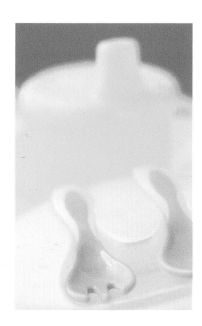

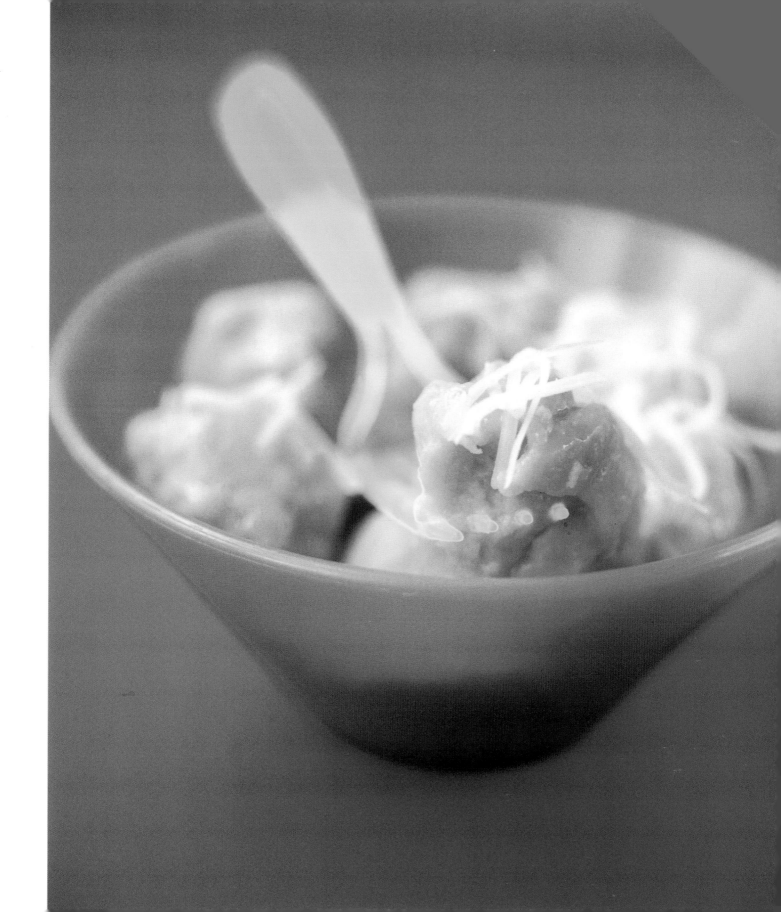

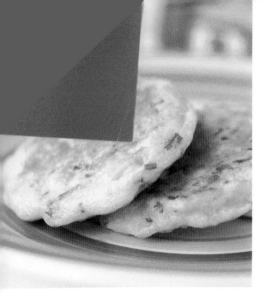

SWEETCORN GRIDDLE CAKES

Sweetcorn is a particularly sweet variety of maize, and the process of canning makes it even sweeter, so it is a popular vegetable with many children. These savoury cakes are quick and simple to make and can be cooked on a griddle or in a frying pan. They go down a treat either on their own, or served as an accompaniment to chicken or fish.

4 fresh corn-on-the-cob, cooked (see tip box), or 375 g (12 oz) canned sweetcorn, drained

2 tablespoons cornflour

2 tablespoons polenta flour

small pinch of chilli powder (optional)

2 large eggs, beaten

small bunch of chives, or 4 spring onions, finely chopped

pinch each of salt and pepper (optional)

corn oil, for frying

• If using fresh corn cobs, cook in boiling water for 10-15 minutes. Drain and, when cool enough to handle, hold upright and strip the kernels with downward strokes of a sharp knife.

Put the cornflour, polenta flour, chilli powder, salt and pepper (if using), in a bowl and mix well. Stir in the eggs and chives or spring onions, then the corn kernels.

Heat 2 teaspoons of oil in a large non-stick frying pan, or griddle. Put 4 tablespoons of the corn mixture into the pan, well apart, and flatten slightly. Cook for 4 minutes, then turn and cook for a further 2 minutes. Remove and drain on kitchen paper. Keep warm while cooking the remaining mixture.

Serve with homemade tomato ketchup (see page 36), if you like.

BONUS POINTS
• Sweetcorn offers a good helping of fibre and protein.

OKAY FOR UNDER-ONES?
Omit the salt.

4-6 months Not suitable. See pages 16-19 for other ideas.

6-9 months Liquidize some of a griddle cake with a little milk or water or, once your baby can chew, cut it up small and moisten with a little milk or water.

9-12 months Either cut the food up small, or give your baby a piece to hold.

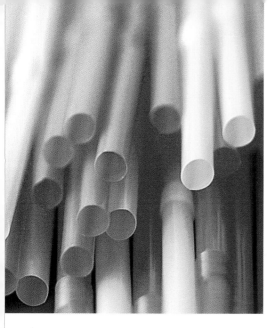

GOTTA LOTTA BOTTLE

Homemade milk shakes are delicious as they bring out the natural flavour and sweetness of fruit. For over-ones, you could sweeten them further if you wish, with a little honey. And you can make them even creamier by adding a spoonful of yogurt or ice cream.

Make the milk shakes one at a time. Put the ingredients, including the yogurt or ice cream (if using), into a blender, and whizz for 30 seconds, or until smooth. Pour into a tall glass.

Add ice cubes and decorate with mint leaves if you like. Pop in 1 or 2 thick drinking straws.

For each milk shake:

175 ml (6 fl oz) full-fat milk

1 teaspoon clear honey (optional)

50 g (2 oz) banana, strawberries, mango, blueberries or blackcurrants

1 tablespoon vanilla ice cream or creamy yogurt (optional)

ice cubes, to serve (optional)

mint leaves, to decorate (optional)

BONUS POINTS

• Milk is rich in protein (for growth and repair) and calcium (especially good for bones, teeth and nerves).
• The various fruits contain antioxidant vitamins, minerals and plant pigments, as well as other helpful 'phyto (plant) nutrients'.

OKAY FOR UNDER-ONES?

4-6 months Not suitable. Instead give some mashed banana, or blend blueberries with a little milk or water.

6-12 months Omit the honey; don't add ice cream or sweetened yogurt. Use full-fat milk. Give your baby no more than 50 ml (2 fl oz) and then not instead of a breast or bottle feed, which should be a baby's main source of milk.

• If preferred, use semi-skimmed milk for children over 2 years of age.
• A milk shake flavoured with blackcurrants needs to be sweetened with a little honey; therefore it isn't suitable for under-ones.

FISH STIR-FRY

White fish is an excellent food for babies – and for older children and adults too. The subtle flavours from the mild chilli sauce, orange juice and vegetables make this a delicious stir-fry, and it's very quick to prepare.

375 g (12 oz) fresh cod or haddock fillets, skinned

2 teaspoons cornflour

75 ml (3 fl oz) freshly squeezed orange juice

1 tablespoon mild sweet chilli sauce

3 medium carrots

3-4 spring onions

4 Chinese leaves or spring greens

1 red pepper, halved, cored and deseeded

200 g (7 oz) medium egg noodles

3 tablespoons vegetable oil

75 g (3 oz) frozen peas

1 tablespoon toasted sesame seeds (optional)

Cut the fish into small chunks and toss in the cornflour to coat. Mix any remaining cornflour with the orange juice and chilli sauce. Shred the carrots, spring onions, Chinese leaves or greens and red pepper, using the shredder attachment of a food processor. Alternatively slice the vegetables very thinly.

Cook the egg noodles in a pan of boiling water according to the packet directions.

Heat the oil in a large frying pan or wok. Add the shredded vegetables and stir-fry for about 3 minutes, until softened but still retaining their texture; remove with a slotted spoon and set aside. Add the fish to the pan and stir-fry for 3 minutes until cooked through. Return the vegetables to the pan. Add the peas and chilli sauce mixture, and heat through for 1 minute, stirring gently.

Drain the noodles and transfer to serving bowls. Spoon the stir-fry on top and serve scattered with sesame seeds if using.

BONUS POINTS
• This stir-fry is packed with protein (for growth), vitamin B (for healthy nerves) and vitamin C (for good resistance to infection).
• The peas and noodles supply slow-release energy.

OKAY FOR UNDER-ONES?
4-6 months Not suitable. Give a 4 month-old some mashed carrots or blended Chinese leaves or spring greens instead. At 5 months you could add a little mashed fish or peas, suitably moistened with water, expressed breast milk or formula, or homemade chicken or vegetable stock.
6-12 months Omit sesame seeds. Blend the food for younger babies who can't cope with lumps; cut up the noodles and mash the fish for older babies.

• If you're short of time, use a bag of ready prepared stir-fry vegetables from the supermarket.
• Frozen fish fillets make a good alternative to fresh fish.

FISH PIE

This tasty pie is good enough to convert the most reluctant fish eater. The light texture of the fish and smooth root mash contrast well with the crisp breadcrumb topping, and the herbs impart a wonderful fragrance.

500 g (1 lb) potatoes, cut into large chunks

500 g (1 lb) swede, cut into large chunks

625 g (1¼ lb) fresh cod, haddock, ling or salmon fillets

450 ml (¾ pint) milk

25 g (1 oz) butter

1 leek, trimmed and finely sliced

25 g (1 oz) plain flour

75 g (3 oz) bread, crusts removed

2 teaspoons chopped fresh parsley or chervil

black pepper

Put the potatoes and swede in a pan, add water to cover and bring to the boil. Cook for 15-20 minutes, or until soft. At the same time, steam the fish fillets in a steamer over the vegetables, or poach in water to cover for 12 minutes.

Drain the potatoes and swede thoroughly. Mash with a third of the milk, and pepper to taste.

Melt the butter in a pan, add the leek and cook for 5-6 minutes, until softened. Stir in the flour and cook for 1 minute, then slowly add the rest of the milk, stirring over the heat, to make a smooth sauce. Take off the heat.

Flake the cooked fish with a fork, then add to the sauce. Spread the mixture in the base of a greased shallow ovenproof dish.

Put the bread and herbs in a blender or food processor and pulse briefly, to make herby breadcrumbs.

Spoon the mash over the fish, then scatter the herby breadcrumbs on top. Bake in a preheated oven at 190°C (375°F) Gas Mark 5 for 25-30 minutes, until golden brown. Serve with peas, spring greens or green cabbage.

BONUS POINTS
• Fish is rich in protein, and also low in saturated fats.

OKAY FOR UNDER-ONES?
4-6 months Not suitable. Give a little cooked potato and/or swede, mashed with some milk or water.

6-12 months Check carefully for bones. Blend some of the fish and vegetable mash with a little milk or water. Once your baby can chew, cut the fish and vegetables up small and mash with some of the topping.

> • If you do not have time to shop for fresh fish, use frozen fish fillets or canned salmon instead.

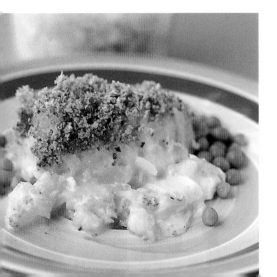

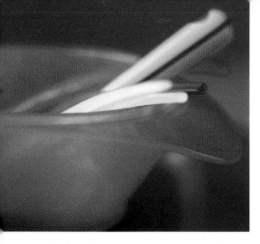

COCONUT MACKEREL WITH SWEET POTATO

Coconut gives fish a delightful sweetness and a distinctive nuttiness, and this tempting recipe treats your family to a taste of the South Pacific.

oil, for brushing

1 kg (2 lb) sweet potato, peeled and cut into 1 cm (½ inch) slices

125 g (4 oz) spinach leaves, roughly torn

750 g (1½ lb) mackerel fillets, skinned

400 g (13 oz) can coconut milk

300 ml (½ pint) water

black pepper

Brush the base of a heavy-based flameproof casserole with oil, then cover with the sweet potato slices. Lay the spinach over the potato, then place the mackerel fillets on top. Season lightly with pepper and pour on the coconut milk and water.

Slowly bring to the boil on the hob. Cover and transfer the casserole to a preheated oven at 180°C (350°F) Gas Mark 4. Cook for 1 hour, or until the liquid is absorbed and the sweet potato is tender: check after 45 minutes that there is still some liquid; if not add a little extra water, otherwise the sweet potatoes may stick to the bottom.

Serve accompanied by peas or green beans, and roasted sweet red and yellow peppers if you like.

BONUS POINTS

• Children in particular love the sweetness of coconut and sweet potato, and this is a good way of encouraging them to eat fish.

• Mackerel is an oily fish, which means it is rich in the omega-3 fats that many people today lack; these help balance the saturated fats in the coconut milk.

OKAY FOR UNDER-ONES?

4-6 months Not suitable. Instead, give some cooked sweet potato mashed with a little milk or water.

6-12 months Check carefully for any small bones, then blend with a little milk or water. Once your baby can chew, cut the food up small and moisten if necessary with a little water or milk.

• For extra flavour, add 1 lemon grass stalk, bruised; 2.5 cm (1 inch) piece of fresh root ginger, peeled and grated; and ¼ teaspoon ground cumin seeds.

• Coconut contains quite a lot of saturated fats, so you may wish to cut down on other saturated fats (in red meat, butter, cheese, etc) that day.

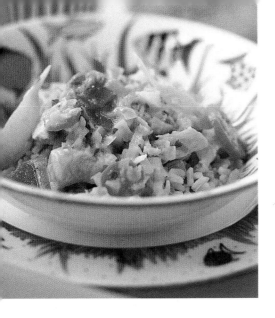

CHICKEN CASSEROLE

A chicken casserole is something you can assemble quickly, pop into the oven, then forget about while you do something else. As it cooks, the wonderful aroma from the oven will stimulate everyone's appetite. An advantage of this casserole is that it is easily adapted for babies.

4 chicken quarters or breasts, or
   8 chicken thighs or drumsticks
2 tablespoons plain flour
2 tablespoons corn or rapeseed
   (canola) oil
2 leeks, trimmed and chopped
2 carrots, sliced
1-2 garlic cloves, crushed
3-4 turnips, cut into 2.5 cm (1 inch)
   chunks, or 6-8 whole baby turnips
2 tablespoons small red lentils
2 teaspoons chopped fresh mixed herbs
   (such as parsley, oregano and thyme)
   or 1 teaspoon dried
1 litre (1¾ pints) chicken stock (see page
   84) or water
black pepper
75 ml (3 fl oz) single cream, or crème
   fraîche (optional)

• This dish freezes well, so you might like to make double the quantity and freeze half for another occasion.
• To lower the fat content, use skinless chicken pieces and don't add cream or crème fraîche.

Toss the chicken pieces in the flour to coat evenly, shaking off the excess.

Heat the oil in a heavy-based flameproof casserole, add the leeks and carrots, and cook gently for 7-8 minutes, stirring occasionally, until softened; remove with a slotted spoon and set aside.

Add the chicken pieces and garlic to the casserole and cook for 8-10 minutes, turning the chicken occasionally to brown on all sides.

Add the turnips, lentils, herbs and pepper, then return the sautéed vegetables to the casserole. Pour in the chicken stock or water and bring to the boil.

Cover the casserole and cook in a preheated oven at 180°C (350°F) Gas Mark 4 for 1¼ hours. Remove from the oven and stir in the cream or crème fraîche (if using).

Serve accompanied by boiled rice (preferably brown), or steamed or baked sweet potatoes, and peas.

BONUS POINTS
• A casserole like this is an excellent way of incorporating more vegetables into a meal. As they cook, the vegetables take on some of the flavour of the chicken, which makes them more appealing to children.
• Lentils help to thicken the liquid around the chicken and vegetables. They also provide slowly absorbed carbohydrates, which help prevent energy levels flagging.

OKAY FOR UNDER-ONES?
Remove any bones. Use salt-free stock.
4-6 months Omit the flour. Blend some of the cooked carrot and/or turnip with a little milk or water. For a baby over 5 months, blend some chicken and moisten with some of the cooking liquid.
6-10 months Blend some of the vegetables, chicken and cooking liquid. Once your baby can cope, mince the chicken and mash the vegetables with some of the liquid.
10-12 months Cut the food up small.

CHICKEN RISI BISI

2 large boneless, skinless chicken
   breasts
25 g (1 oz) butter
1 tablespoon olive or rapeseed (canola)
   oil
1 onion, chopped
1 garlic clove, crushed
400 g (13 oz) arborio or other risotto rice,
   (preferably brown)
1.2 litres (2 pints) hot vegetable stock (see
   page 51) or chicken stock (see page 84)
150 g (5 oz) mangetout, cut diagonally
   into 2.5 cm (1 inch) lengths
50 g (2 oz) Parmesan or Cheddar
   cheese, grated (optional)

• You'd make a 'classic' risotto by
adding the stock to the pan a little
at a time, stirring continuously, and
adding more stock once it's
absorbed. My method is simpler,
but the results are equally good.

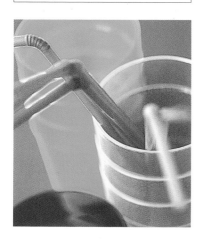

Visit Venice and you'll see 'risi e bisi' – rice and peas – on the menu of nearly every street café. Add some chicken and you have a flavourful risotto popular with all children. Vary the vegetables according to taste – chopped carrots, ordinary peas, broccoli, broad beans and sweetcorn are all suitable.

Cut the chicken into small chunks. Melt the butter with the oil in a large, heavy-based saucepan. Add the chicken and fry gently for about 5 minutes until cooked through. Remove with a slotted spoon.

Add the onion and garlic to the pan and fry gently for 2 minutes. Stir in the rice and cook for 1 minute.

Add a ladleful of the stock; cook, stirring, until absorbed. Add about two thirds of the remaining stock and cook gently, stirring frequently. Once the stock is almost absorbed and the rice is nearly tender, return the chicken to the pan and add the mangetout and remaining stock.

Cook for a further 5 minutes or until the rice is tender, adding a little more stock if the mixture becomes dry. Stir in the cheese (if using), to serve.

BONUS POINTS
• The chicken, rice and peas together are a good source of vitamin B, protein and long-lasting energy.
• Brown rice contains three times as much fibre, twice as much zinc, and six times as much magnesium and vitamin E as white rice.

OKAY FOR UNDER-ONES?
4-6 months Not suitable.
6-12 months Blend the food for younger babies who can't cope with lumps; by about 10 months most babies can chew chicken if it's cut up very small.

Chicken stock
Put a small whole chicken or 4 chicken pieces in a large pan with 1 onion, quartered; 2 carrots, quartered; 1 celery stick, cut into lengths; 1 garlic clove, peeled; and some pepper. Simmer gently, partially covered, for 1½ hours, or 1 hour if using chicken pieces. Strain the stock and use as required.

Freeze stock in an ice-cube tray so you always have some to hand to moisten a baby's food. Or freeze a larger quantity in a suitable rigid container.

You can buy fresh chilled chicken stock from selected supermarkets and butchers. Check it has no added salt if you are giving it to a baby under one.

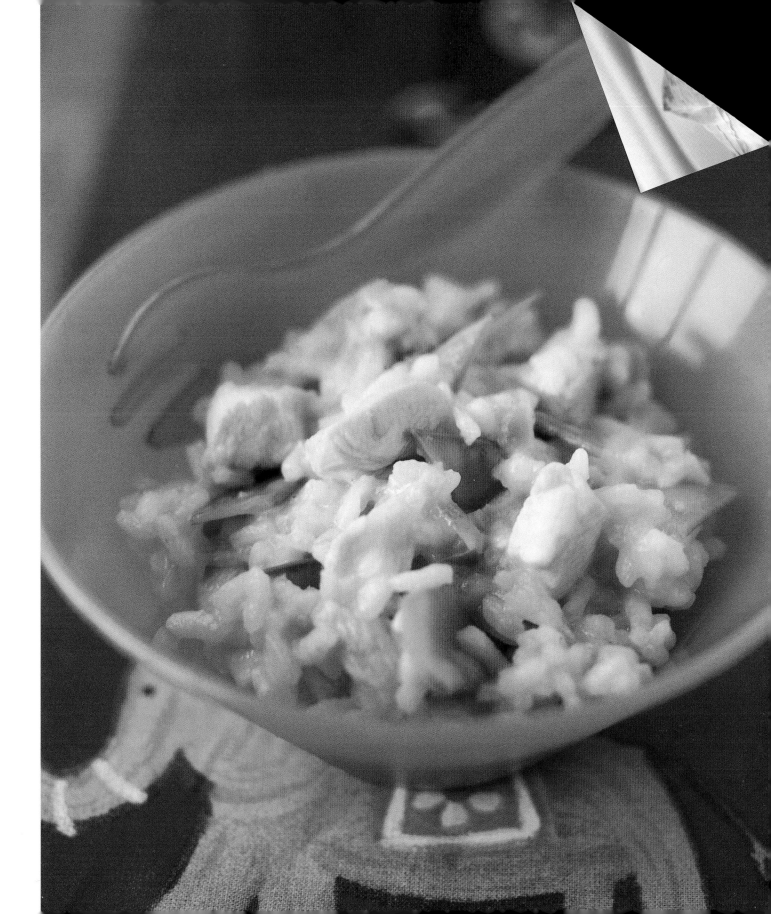

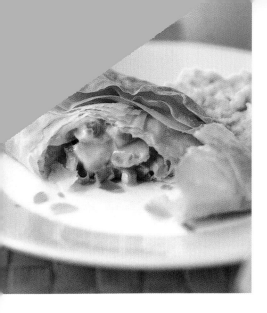

CHICKEN & VEGETABLE PIES

There's something about wrapping food in pastry that makes it more appealing, and children of all ages love these tasty filo pies. If you have any leftover, pop one into your child's packed lunch box the following day.
Makes 10 small pies

2 large boneless, skinless chicken breasts

50 g (2 oz) butter

1 large leek, trimmed and chopped

150 g (5 oz) carrots, thinly sliced

2 teaspoons plain flour

200 ml (7 fl oz) fresh chicken stock, preferably homemade (see page 84)

100 g (3½ oz) French beans, sliced

4 tablespoons double cream

175 g (6 oz) ready-made filo pastry

• These individual chicken pies make good freezer standbys. Freeze the uncooked pies in a rigid container. Defrost at room temperature for 2-3 hours, or overnight in the refrigerator, then bake as above.

Cut the chicken into small cubes. Melt 25 g (1 oz) of the butter in a large frying pan. Add the chicken and fry for 3 minutes until lightly browned. Add the leek and carrots and fry for 2 minutes until the leeks have wilted. Stir in the flour.

Stir in the stock, then add the French beans and bring to the boil, stirring. Cover and cook gently for 5 minutes. Stir in the cream and leave to cool.

Melt the remaining butter. Cut the pastry into thirty 13 cm (5 inch) squares. Lightly brush one filo square with butter, cover with another square and brush with butter. Add a third square and brush the edges with butter. Place a heaped dessertspoon of the chicken mixture in the centre. Bring up the corners of the pastry to meet over the filling and pinch the edges together to form an envelope shape. Repeat with the remaining filling and pastry to make 10 pies in total.

Place the pies on a lightly greased baking sheet and brush with the remaining butter. Bake in a preheated oven at 200°C (400°F) Gas Mark 6 for 15-20 minutes, or until golden brown. Serve with creamy mashed potato and carrots, or a tomato salad.

BONUS POINT
• The vegetables inside each little pie help towards one of the 5 daily helpings of vegetables and fruit recommended for over-twos.

OKAY FOR UNDER-ONES?
4-6 months Not suitable. Instead, give some carrot, leek or French beans, mashed or blended and suitably moistened.
6-12 months Blend the food for younger babies who can't yet cope with lumps. By about 10 months most babies will manage to chew diced chicken, so you can cut the pies into small pieces.

BARBECUED SPARE RIBS

Sweet, succulent spare ribs roasted in the oven are exceptionally yummy and easy to eat with fingers – remember to provide napkins. These ribs are equally good served with vegetables or salad. You can also cook them on the barbecue when the weather permits.

2 tablespoons tomato purée, or tomato ketchup (preferably homemade, see page 36)

2 tablespoons redcurrant jelly

2 teaspoons soy sauce (optional)

2 teaspoons chopped fresh sage or parsley

2 garlic cloves, crushed

8 large pork spare ribs

black pepper

In a large shallow bowl, mix the tomato purée or tomato ketchup with the redcurrant jelly, soy sauce (if using), sage or parsley, garlic and pepper. Add the spare ribs and turn to coat well with the marinade. Cover the bowl with clingfilm and place in the refrigerator. Leave to marinate for at least 1 hour (preferably overnight).

Transfer the ribs and marinade to a roasting tin. Bake in a preheated oven at 180°C (350°F) Gas Mark 4 for 40-45 minutes, or until well cooked, then pour off the fat.

Serve hot, accompanied by baked potatoes in their jackets or brown rice and a green vegetable, or a salad.

BONUS POINTS
• Pork is rich in B vitamins (for healthy nerves) and zinc (for immunity, and healthy skin and mucous membranes).

OKAY FOR UNDER-ONES?
Not suitable. See pages 16-19 for other first food ideas.

• If the spare ribs are very fatty; limit your family's intake of fatty food – particularly foods high in saturated fat – for the rest of the day.

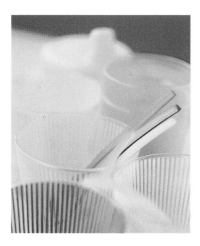

87

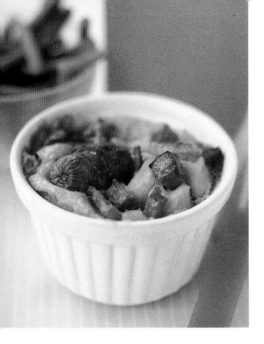

TOAD 'N ROOTS IN THE HOLE

Tasty roasted root vegetables are incorporated into this delicious variation of traditional toad-in-the-hole. Roasting brings out the full sweet, earthy flavour of roots, such as swede, beetroot and carrots.

375 g (12 oz) raw beetroot, scrubbed, or swede, peeled

2 carrots

2 onions, quartered

3 tablespoons corn or rapeseed (canola) oil

8 sausages

8 rashers of streaky bacon

125 g (4 oz) plain flour

1 egg

300 ml (½ pint) milk

salt (optional) and black pepper

Cut the beetroot or swede and carrots into 4 cm (1½ inch) chunks. Put in a roasting tin with the quartered onions, drizzle with the oil and toss to coat. Roast in a preheated oven at 190°C (375°F) Gas Mark 5 for 25 minutes.

Meanwhile, prick the sausages with a fork and wrap a bacon rasher around each one.

Remove the roasting tin from the oven, turn the vegetables, add the bacon-wrapped sausages and turn them to coat with oil. Roast for a further 10 minutes.

Meanwhile, make the batter. Put the flour into a bowl and stir in the egg, half the milk, a pinch of salt (if using) and a little pepper. Whisk in the remaining milk until smooth.

Turn the sausages and spread them and the vegetables evenly in the roasting tin. Pour in the batter, return to the oven and bake for a further 40 minutes until the batter is well risen and crisp. Serve with peas or cabbage, and baked beans if you like.

BONUS POINTS
• Milk offers plenty of calcium (for strong bones and teeth), as well as protein (for growth and healing).
• This is a good all-in-one choice for those who are reluctant to eat vegetables.

OKAY FOR UNDER-ONES?
4-6 months Not suitable. Instead, steam some carrot or swede and blend with a little milk or water.
6-12 months Omit salt, bacon and sausages unless salt-free sausages are available. Blend the cooked vegetables and batter with a little milk or water. Or, once your baby can chew, cut up small and moisten, if necessary, with milk or water.

• Use good quality butcher's-style sausages and experiment with different flavours.
• For a vegetarian option, omit the sausages and increase the vegetables, including other varieties, such as parsnips and leeks, cut into chunks.

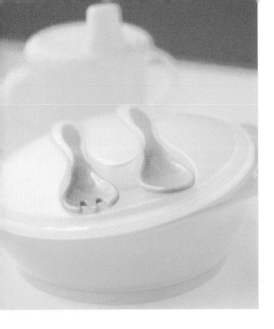

COUSCOUS

Made of coarse semolina, couscous is traditionally steamed over a pan of lamb and vegetable stew and lends its name to the resulting dish. It soaks up the flavours of the fragrant simmering stew to delicious effect. Couscous is a popular staple in north African countries, including Morocco, where it originates from.

125 g (4 oz) dried chickpeas, soaked overnight in cold water

500g (1 lb) lamb neck fillet, trimmed of fat

2 tablespoons olive oil

2 Spanish onions, quartered

pinch of powdered saffron

pinch of ground ginger (optional)

pinch of ground cinnamon (optional)

600 ml (1 pint) water

500 g (1 lb) couscous (not 'instant')

4 tomatoes, quartered

375 g (12 oz) pumpkin, cut into 2.5 cm (1 inch) chunks

3 carrots, cut into 1 cm (½ inch) slices

2 courgettes, cut into 1 cm (½ inch) slices

50 g (2 oz) raisins

black pepper

25 g (1 oz) butter, in pieces (optional)

• Instead of dried chickpeas, you may prefer to use a 425 g (14 oz) can chickpeas, drained, or fresh or frozen broad beans; add to the stew with the carrots and other vegetables.

Drain the chickpeas and simmer in water to cover for 1 hour; drain. Line a perforated steamer with muslin. Cut the lamb into 2.5 cm (1 inch) chunks.

Put the oil, chickpeas, lamb, onions, spices (if using), and pepper in the bottom of the steamer pan. Add the water, bring to the boil, cover and simmer for 1 hour.

Meanwhile, put the couscous into a large fine sieve and rinse under cold running water, stirring with your fingers. Spread the couscous out in a shallow tin, leave for 15 minutes, then break up any lumps with your fingers.

Put the couscous into the muslin-lined steamer. Place this over the steamer pan, but don't cover. Simmer the stew for 20 minutes, then remove the steamer containing the couscous. Cover the pan and continue to simmer the stew for a further 20 minutes, adding more water if necessary.

Meanwhile, turn the couscous into the shallow tin again, stir in 300 ml (½ pint) of cold water, and break up any lumps with your fingers or a fork.

Stir the tomatoes, pumpkin, carrots, courgettes and raisins into the stew. Return the couscous to the muslin-lined steamer, replace over the stew and simmer uncovered, for 30 minutes, adding more water if needed.

Pile the couscous on to a serving dish and fork in the butter (if using). Make a well in the centre and spoon in the meat and vegetables to serve.

BONUS POINTS
• Couscous supplies a generous helping of starchy carbohydrate, and is a good vehicle for providing children with some of the vegetables they need each day.

OKAY FOR UNDER-ONES?
4-6 months Not suitable. Give a 4 month-old some pumpkin, and/or carrot, removed from the broth and puréed with milk or water. A 5 month-old can have a little lamb, blended with some of the vegetables and a little water.
6-12 months Blend the food or, once your baby can chew, cut it up small. Give for lunch rather than supper if chickpeas make your baby windy.

MAGIC MINCE

1 onion, roughly chopped

3 medium carrots, roughly chopped

2 celery sticks, roughly chopped

2 courgettes, roughly chopped

4 tablespoons olive oil

500 g (1 lb) lean minced lamb, beef or pork

2 garlic cloves, chopped

2-3 teaspoons ground paprika

300 ml (½ pint) fresh chicken stock, preferably homemade (see page 84)

400 g (13 oz) can chickpeas, rinsed and drained (see tip box)

100 g (3½ oz) ready-to-eat prunes, chopped

• A useful recipe to make in bulk and freeze in convenient portions.

• Chick peas canned in brine are unsuitable for under-ones, but cooked dried chickpeas, kidney beans or lentils can be substituted. Remember to pre-soak dried pulses.

This mildly spiced mince is enlivened with chopped prunes and chickpeas, but you could easily substitute dried apricots or sultanas for the prunes, and lentils, red kidney beans or butter beans for the chickpeas, if you prefer. Finely chopping plenty of vegetables in the food processor before combining them with meat is a great way to disguise their appearance and encourage children who are fussy about eating them.

Put the onion, carrots and celery in a food processor and pulse until finely chopped. Take out and repeat with the courgettes.

Heat 2 tablespoons of the oil in a large pan. Add the vegetables and fry quickly for 5 minutes; remove with a slotted spoon. Add the remaining oil to the pan and fry the minced meat with the garlic for 5 minutes, breaking it up with a wooden spoon.

Return the vegetables to the pan, and add the paprika, stock, chickpeas and prunes. Bring to the boil, cover with a lid and cook gently for about 30 minutes until thickened and pulpy.

Serve with pasta, steamed couscous, rice, mashed potatoes, or with a mashed potato topping; plus steamed broccoli, cabbage or French beans.

BONUS POINTS

• Chickpeas provide slow-release carbohydrates that help keep a child feeling full of energy for a longer period of time.

• Prunes supply a touch of sweetness and also help guard against constipation.

OKAY FOR UNDER-ONES?

Use cooked dried chickpeas, beans or lentils rather than those canned in water with added salt.

4-6 months Not suitable.

6-12 months Blend for younger babies who can't cope with lumps, and cut the vegetables up very small for older babies.

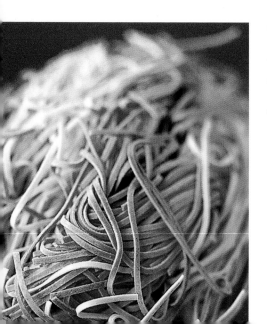

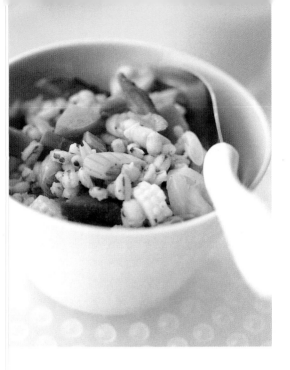

BARLEY POT

Barley is rarely used, yet it is versatile, nutritious and sustaining. Don't confuse pot barley with pearl barley. Both grains have had their outer husk removed, but pot barley grains are otherwise whole, whereas 'pearling' (or polishing) barley removes most of the bran and germ, along with a good deal of the protein, vitamin B, calcium and iron. Not only is pot barley far more nutritious, it also has a good chewy texture and nutty flavour.

375 g (12 oz) pot barley, (preferably pre-soaked in cold water for 6-8 hours)

50 g (2 oz) butter

250 g (8 oz) bacon steaks, cut into strips (optional)

4-6 spring onions, chopped

2 carrots, chopped

3-4 baby corn, chopped

50 g (2 oz) French beans, cut into short lengths

2 teaspoons wholegrain mustard (optional)

black pepper

1 tablespoon molasses (optional)

2 teaspoons dried mixed herbs

300 ml (½ pint) fresh chicken stock, preferably homemade (see page 84)

600 ml (1 pint) water (approximately)

Melt the butter in a heavy-based casserole dish. Add the bacon (if using), spring onions and carrots, and cook for 5 minutes, stirring frequently.

Stir in the barley, baby corn, French beans, mustard (if using) and pepper. Cook, stirring frequently, for 2 minutes.

Add the molasses (if using), mixed herbs, stock and water, and bring to the boil. Cover and cook in a preheated oven at 180°C (350°F) Gas Mark 4 for 1½ hours, checking from time to time that the mixture isn't becoming dry, and adding more water if necessary.

Serve with steamed shredded Savoy or other green cabbage.

BONUS POINTS
• Pot barley's soluble fibre helps lower the cholesterol level and steady the blood sugar for several hours. Barley also contains anti-viral agents, called protease inhibitors.
• Pot barley also supplies protein (for growth and repair), vitamin B (for nerves), calcium (for bones, teeth and nerves) and iron (for haemoglobin).

OKAY FOR UNDER-ONES?
Omit bacon. Use salt-free stock. For older babies, chicken or lamb can be used.
4-6 months Omit mustard. Take out some cooked barley and blend with a little milk or water. A baby of 5 months can have some chicken blended with a little milk or water instead, or if familiar with that taste, some chicken and barley together.
6-10 months Use only 1 teaspoon of mustard. Blend with a little milk or water, or give the unblended barley on its own.
10-12 months If including chicken or lamb instead of bacon, cut up small.

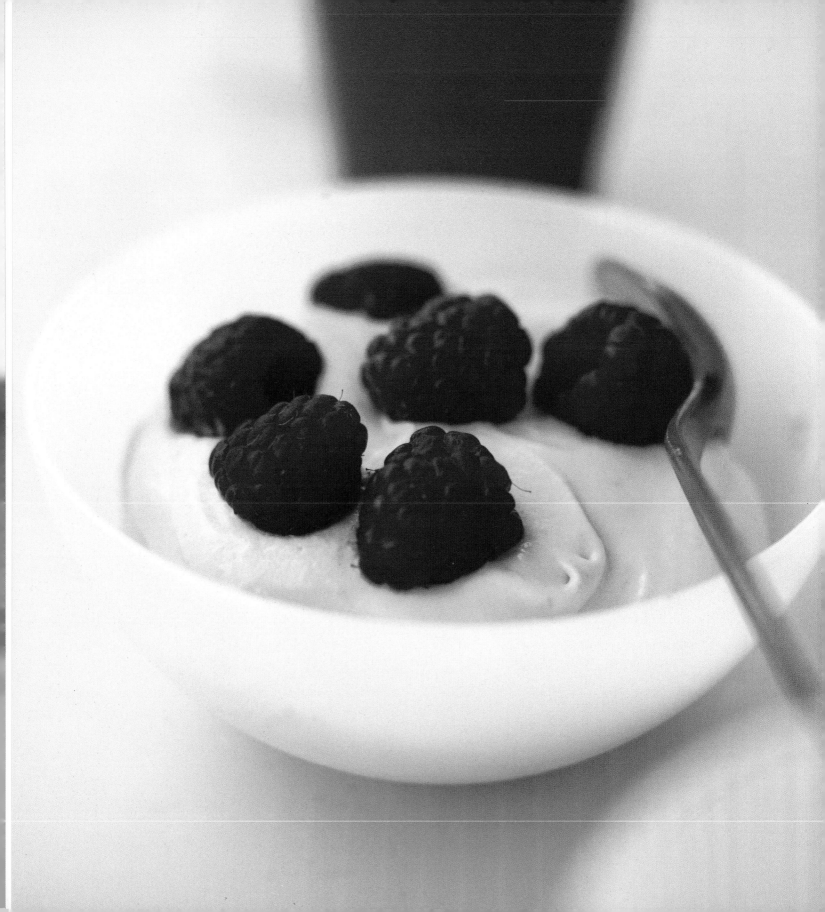

What's for Pud?

Fresh fruit is nature's own dessert and is popular with most children if it's perfectly ripe and ready to eat. Yogurt is another excellent healthy choice, though some children and adults prefer to round off a meal with something more savoury, like a little cheese. For the occasional special dessert, choose from the mouth-watering ideas in this chapter, such as Raspberry Fool, Baked Plum Custard and irresistible Chocolate Puddle Pud.

CREAMY RASPBERRY FOOL

Raspberries are one of life's great treats, with their deep rose colour and intense flavour. Occasionally raspberries are so sweet they need no extra sugar, but they usually require a little (ideally not for under-ones). *Serves 6*

200 g (7 oz) fresh raspberries

2-3 tablespoons icing sugar (preferably unrefined)

5 tablespoons double cream

200 g (7 oz) fromage frais

Set aside 25 g (1 oz) of the raspberries. Purée the rest in a blender or food processor, then press through a sieve into a bowl to remove the seeds. Stir in the icing sugar to taste.

Whip the cream in a separate bowl until thickened, then fold in the fromage frais. Add the raspberry purée and beat again until smooth and slightly thickened. Taste for sweetness.

Spoon into small serving bowls and chill until required. Scatter with the reserved raspberries to serve.

BONUS POINTS
• Raspberries are a good source of fibre and plant pigments.
• Fromage frais provides a useful amount of protein and calcium.

OKAY FOR UNDER-ONES?
4-6 months Not suitable. Give some sieved raspberries instead.
6-12 months Omit the icing sugar. Don't be alarmed to see raspberry pips in your baby's nappy, as they pass through intact.

• For over-twos you can use half-fat fromage frais.
• To make a frozen dessert, freeze this fool in little plastic tubs or ice lolly tubes.

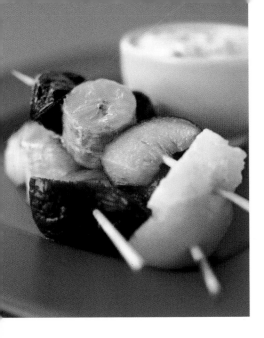

FRUIT KEBABS

Fruit kebabs look wonderful, although on no account should you let your children use them for an impromptu sword fight! Take the fruit off the skewers before serving to under-fives, and supervise older children. Choose a selection of whatever fruits are available, and encourage children to put together their own combinations.

For the coating, combine the ingredients in a large bowl. Add the prepared fruit and toss with your hands to coat in the mixture.

Thread the fruits alternately on to short bamboo skewers and lay on a baking tray. Place under a preheated grill for 2-3 minutes until browned, then carefully turn the kebabs over and brown on the other side for 2 minutes.

Leave the kebabs to cool a little before serving, with Greek yogurt or crème fraîche.

BONUS POINTS
• Fruit is rich in antioxidant plant pigments (which help protect body cells from damage) and in fibre (which helps guard against constipation and maintain a healthy blood-cholesterol level).
• Figs are particularly good, because they provide three times as much calcium as the other fruits, along with plenty of phosphorus to help the body absorb that calcium.

OKAY FOR UNDER-ONES?
Remove fruit from skewers and keep skewers well away from babies and toddlers.
4-6 months Not suitable. Blend some stewed eating apple, pear, peach or apricot with milk; or mash some banana with milk.
6-9 months Give some stewed eating apple, pear, apricot, or prunes; or some fresh pear, apricot, peach or banana, sweetened with a little fruit juice. Mash the fruit, unless your baby can cope with finger food, then give slices of raw apple, pear, peach or apricot, or pieces of banana or pineapple. Serve with yogurt rather than crème fraîche.
9-12 months Give the above fruits, mashed, cut into little pieces, or served as finger foods, with yogurt.

Choose 4-6 of the following:

1 eating apple, quartered and cored

1 firm pear, quartered and cored

1 firm banana, cut into 4 chunks

8 large prunes, stoned

2 fresh or dried figs, halved

2 slices fresh pineapple, peeled, cored
    and halved, or 2 pineapple
    rings canned in natural juice, halved

1 firm peach, halved and stoned

2 apricots, halved and stoned

Coating:

grated rind and juice of 1 lemon

2 tablespoons maple syrup

2 tablespoons hazelnut or walnut oil

• If preferred, you can grill the fruits without coating them first: they won't look as shiny and will taste less sweet, but have the benefit of no added sugar.

FRESH FRUIT SALAD

A fresh fruit dessert is straightforward to prepare, easy for children to eat, and perennially popular. Most fruits are available all year round, but it makes sense to choose homegrown varieties when they are in season, and at their peak of flavour. Try these appealing combinations.

2 oranges
1 apple, cored and chopped
1 pear, cored and chopped
200 ml (7 fl oz) apple juice
1-2 bananas

Peel and segment 1 orange; squeeze the juice from the other one. Put all the ingredients, except the banana, in a large bowl and toss to mix.

Slice the banana and add to the fruit salad just before serving, otherwise it will discolour. Toss to mix.

Serve with yogurt or crème fraîche, or ice cream.

VARIATIONS
Melon and blueberry salad Quarter, deseed, peel and chop 1 small melon. Toss with 175 g (6 oz) fresh blueberries in 300 ml (½ pint) apple juice.

Mango and banana salad Peel and chop 2 ripe mangoes, cutting the flesh away from the stones. Toss the chopped mango with 2 sliced bananas in 300 ml (½ pint) apple and mango juice.

Pear, raspberry and kiwi salad Core and slice 2 fresh ripe pears and mix with 175 g (6 oz) raspberries, 2 sliced kiwi fruit, and 300 ml (½ pint) fruit juice, such as apple and pear, apple and raspberry, red grape, or pineapple juice. (Illustrated left)

BONUS POINTS
• Fresh fruit is laden with plant pigments, vitamin C and other antioxidants, all of which help boost immunity and keep the body fit and well.

OKAY FOR UNDER-ONES?
4-6 months Give some ripe pear, banana, melon, blueberries or mango, mashed with little fruit juice. Or offer some stewed eating apple.
6-9 months As above, or, when a baby is old enough to hold and suck food, give pieces of fruit to eat with their fingers.
9-12 months As above, or, when your baby can chew, give fruit cut up small and mix with a little fruit juice.

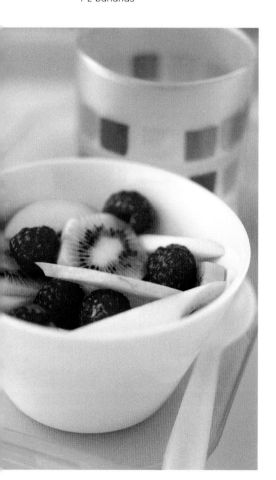

ICED MANGO YOGURT

This creamy, fruity yogurt makes a light, refreshing pud or between-meal treat. Choose mangoes carefully – they are ready to eat if they give slightly when you press them gently. Alternatively, you can use ripe pears or canned mangoes instead. *Serves 8*

100 g (3½ oz) golden caster sugar
75 ml (3 fl oz) water
2 medium ripe mangoes
juice of 1 lemon
500 ml (17 fl oz) Greek yogurt

• This mixture can also be used to make delicious ice lollies for older children. After whisking the partially frozen yogurt ice, pack into 8-10 plastic lolly moulds and freeze overnight until firm. To unmould, briefly hold under hot running water until the mould can be eased away.

Put the sugar and water in a small heavy-based saucepan and heat gently until the sugar dissolves. Leave to cool.

Halve, stone and peel the mangoes. Cut the flesh up roughly and place in a food processor or blender. Add the lemon juice and blend until smooth. Turn into a bowl.

Add the cooled syrup and yogurt to the mango purée and beat well. Transfer to a shallow plastic container and freeze until thickened around the edges, about 2 hours.

Turn the mixture into a bowl and whisk until smooth and thickened. Return to the freezer container. Cover and freeze for at least 2 hours, or overnight until firm.

Transfer to the refrigerator about 30 minutes before serving to soften slightly. Serve the iced yogurt on its own or with a fresh fruit salad.

BONUS POINTS
• Mangoes are a good source of beta-carotene; lemon juice provides vitamin C; and the yogurt adds plenty of protein.

OKAY FOR UNDER-ONES?
4-6 months Not suitable. Give some puréed mango instead.
6-12 months Although not totally unsuitable, it's better not to give babies foods with added sugar. Instead, give some puréed mango mixed with yogurt.

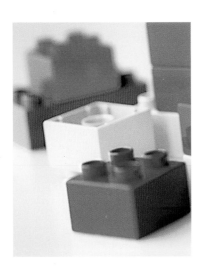

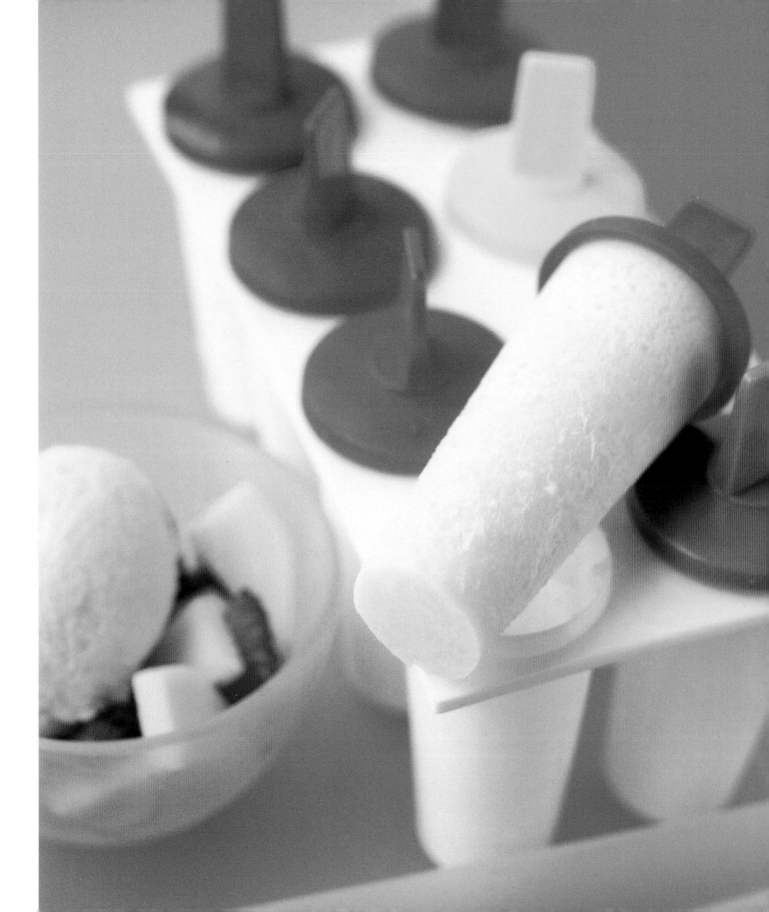

BAKED PLUM CUSTARD

75 g (3 oz) caster sugar

150 ml (¼ pint) water

1 kg (2 lb) red or black plums, stoned

600 ml (1 pint) full-fat milk

4 eggs, plus 4 egg yolks

> • For a hint of spice, add the crushed seeds from 4 green cardamom pods, or a pinch of ground cinnamon to the milk.
> • For a very smooth custard, sieve the cooked plums, to remove the skins.
> • The custard is delicious hot, warm or cold. It will be a little firmer if you cook it ahead of time, because it continues to set on cooling.

This colourful dessert has universal appeal – the custard is rich and creamy, while full-flavoured plums tantalise the tastebuds. An added bonus is that it can be prepared ahead. Pitted cherries can be used instead of plums.

Put the sugar and water in a medium saucepan and heat gently until the sugar is dissolved.

Add the plums, cover and simmer gently, stirring occasionally, for about 5-7 minutes until they are soft. Increase the heat and cook until the water has almost totally evaporated. Set aside 2 tablespoons of the stewed plums in a small bowl.

Heat the milk in a large pan until almost to boiling. Meanwhile, whisk the eggs and egg yolks together in a bowl. Whisk in the hot milk, then pour into a shallow 1.8 litre (3 pint) baking dish. Stir in the plums (from the pan).

Stand the dish in a large roasting tin and surround with boiling water to come halfway up the sides of the dish. Cook in a preheated oven at 170°C (325°F) Gas Mark 3 for 45-50 minutes, or until the custard is just set.

Serve each portion topped with a heaped teaspoon of the reserved stewed plums.

BONUS POINTS
• Eggs are protein-rich and provide useful amounts of vitamin A, B, D and E, especially vitamin B12, which is often lacking in a vegetarian diet; they are also a good source of zinc.

OKAY FOR UNDER-ONES?
4-6 months Not suitable. Instead, give cooked, unsweetened plums, sieved to remove the skins.
6-12 months Cook the plums without added sugar and sieve them before adding to the custard. Or, if your baby can chew, just leave out the sugar. If the plums need extra sweetness, add 1 tablespoon of apple juice to the custard in your baby's bowl.

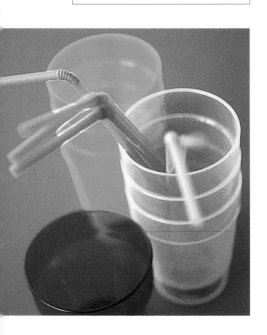

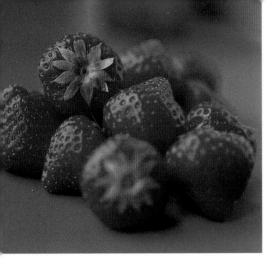

PINK TUBBY CUSTARD

Teletubbies aren't the only ones to enjoy a little dish of pink custard – young children love it and many older children and adults too! This dessert is quick and easy to make but the custard takes time to cool, so make it ahead of time. You can use fresh (or frozen) raspberries instead of fresh strawberries if you like.

4 eggs, plus 1 egg yolk

2 tablespoons caster sugar

600 ml (1 pint) milk

½ teaspoon vanilla extract

250 g (8 oz) strawberries

• You could use a bought carton of fresh custard (from the supermarket chilled cabinet), though it has a more glutinous texture than homemade custard.

Put the whole eggs, egg yolk, sugar and 4 tablespoons of the milk into a heatproof bowl, and whisk thoroughly.

Meanwhile, heat the rest of the milk in a saucepan until lukewarm. Pour on to the whisked eggs, whisking constantly. Stand the bowl over a pan of simmering water and stir the custard with a wooden spoon, until it thickens slightly – enough to thinly coat the back of the spoon. Immediately take the bowl off the heat.

Pour the custard into a cold bowl and stir in the vanilla extract. Cover the surface closely with dampened greaseproof paper to prevent a skin forming and leave to cool.

Purée the strawberries in a blender, then pass the purée through a sieve, to remove the pips.

Serve the custard in bowls, topped with a thick swirl of strawberry purée.

BONUS POINTS

• Milk is a good source of protein (for growth and repair) and calcium (for bones, teeth and healthy nerves).

• Eggs are high in protein. They are a valuable source of vitamin B12 too, particularly for children who don't obtain this vitamin from meat and fish.

• Strawberries are very rich in vitamin C. They also contain pectin, a type of soluble fibre that helps to keep arteries healthy. They may also help prevent viral infections.

OKAY FOR UNDER-ONES?

4-6 months Only give only some of the puréed strawberries.

6-12 months Suitable.

FRUIT CRUMBLE

A good crumble, with its crunchy top and soft inside, moistened from beneath by a soft layer of sweet fruit, makes a wonderful sustaining pudding. Apple and mango is an original combination that appeals to children, but you can vary the fruit according to whatever is available.

2 large cooking apples
1 mango
juice of 1 lemon
125-150 g (4-5 oz) muscovado sugar
200 g (7 oz) plain flour
1 teaspoon baking powder
25 g (1 oz) ground almonds
75 g (3 oz) butter, cut into small pieces
25-50 g (1-2 oz) rolled oats

Peel, core and slice the apples; peel and slice the mango, discarding the stone. Mix the fruit with the lemon juice and 25-50 g (1-2 oz) sugar to taste, in a buttered 1.8 litre (3 pint) pie dish.

Mix the flour, baking powder and ground almonds together in a large bowl. Add the butter and rub in until the mixture resembles fine breadcrumbs. Stir in the 75 g (3 oz) of sugar, plus the oats.

Spread the crumble over the fruit and bake in a preheated oven at 180°C (350°F) Gas Mark 4 for about 30 minutes, or until the top is golden brown. Serve with custard, vanilla ice cream or creamy yogurt.

Variation
Other fruit can be used, such as apples and blackberries; apples and blackcurrants; plums; pears and bananas. You will need 500 g (1 lb) fruit in total; there is no need to add sugar to a filling of pears and bananas.

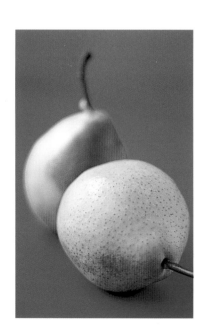

BONUS POINTS
• Fruit is rich in antioxidant vitamins (that help protect body cells from damage) and fibre (which helps prevent constipation and keep arteries healthy).

OKAY FOR UNDER-ONES?
Not suitable.
4-6 months Blend some stewed eating apple with milk.
6-9 months Give some stewed fruit: eating apple; blackcurrants sweetened with a little apple juice; or sieved dessert plums. Mash the fruit and serve with yogurt.
9-12 months As above, or cut up small, or give pieces of raw apple, pear, mango, or banana as finger foods. Serve with yogurt.

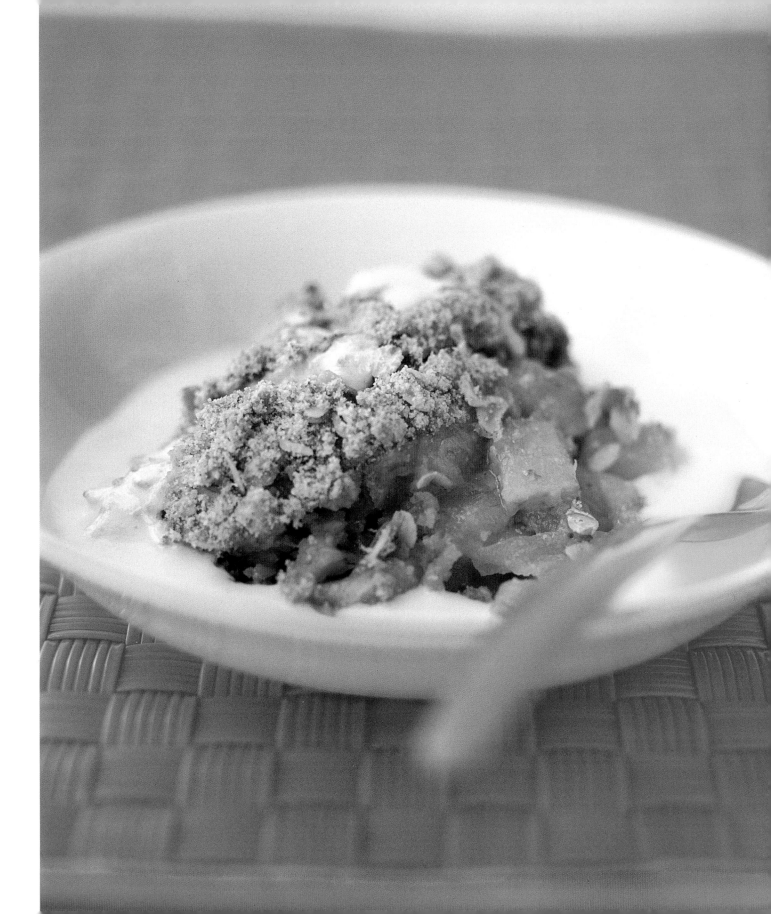

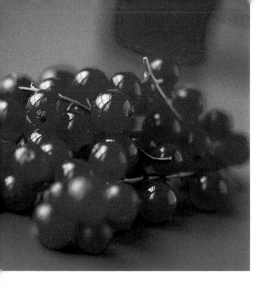

RICE PUDDING WITH FRUIT SAUCE

Most people's idea of rice pudding is of a bland, sweet dessert – or the somewhat artificial taste of canned rice pudding – but this version wins hands down. Originating from Denmark, it is traditionally served chilled with a hot sauce of blueberries, plums, blackberries, or black or redcurrants.

600 ml (1 pint) full-fat milk

125 g (4 oz) white long-grain rice

50 g (2 oz) caster sugar

1 teaspoon vanilla extract

150 ml (¼ pint) whipping cream (optional)

Fruit sauce:

500 g (1 lb) blueberries, stoned plums, blackberries, raspberries, black or redcurrants (or a mixture)

3 tablespoons water

15-25 g (½-1 oz) caster sugar

Bring the milk to the boil in a saucepan, then pour into a 1.8 litre (3 pint) pie dish. Stir in the rice. Bake in a preheated oven at 180°C (350°F) Gas Mark 4 for 20 minutes, or until the milk is absorbed. Stir in the sugar and vanilla extract, then allow to cool. If using cream, whip it until thick, then fold into the pudding. Chill in the refrigerator.

To make the fruit sauce, put the fruit, water and sugar in a pan and cook, stirring occasionally, for 5 minutes or until soft.

Serve the pudding topped with a generous spoonful of the hot fruit sauce.

BONUS POINTS

• Milk is rich in protein (for growth and repair) and calcium (for strong bones and teeth, and proper nerve function).

OKAY FOR UNDER-ONES?

4-6 months Not suitable. Instead give ground (baby) rice; or blended stewed blueberries; or sieved stewed dessert plums; or both rice and fruit if your baby can cope with more than one flavour.

6-12 months Omit the sugar from the rice pudding, and blend if your baby can't yet cope with lumps. Serve with mashed stewed blueberries, blackcurrants or sieved plums, sweetened with a little apple juice if necessary. Or, if your baby can chew, serve raw blueberries or sweet, ripe plums as finger foods.

• Bags of frozen mixed berry fruits are available from supermarkets.

• As an alternative to fruit, you can serve the rice pudding with heated redcurrant jelly, or a red fruit jam, such as cherry or raspberry (ideally a low-sugar version).

• Or omit the fruit sauce and add 50 g (2 oz) of chopped dried apricots, dates or figs to the milk and rice before baking.

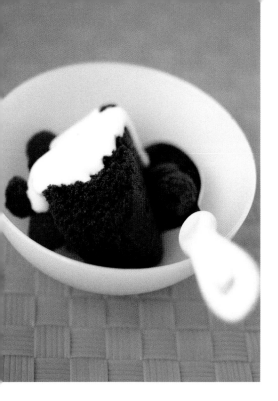

CHOCOLATE PUDDLE PUD

This gorgeous chocolate pudding has the added bonus of a soft centre which forms a puddle of sauce. Serve it after a main course that isn't too rich. Fresh raspberries are an ideal accompaniment.

Put the chocolate and water in a heatproof bowl over a pan of simmering water until melted. Stir until smooth and take the bowl off the heat.

Meanwhile, cream the butter and sugar together in a large bowl until pale and creamy. Gradually beat in the eggs, adding the vanilla extract and 1 tablespoon of the flour with the final addition.

Sift the flour with the cocoa and baking powder over the mixture, then fold in carefully using a large metal spoon, until evenly incorporated. Quickly fold in the melted chocolate alternately with the milk or water.

Spoon into a buttered 1.8 litre (3 pint) pie dish. Bake in a preheated oven at 180°C (350°F) Gas Mark 4 for 30 minutes.

Serve at once, accompanied by fresh raspberries (or defrosted frozen ones); yogurt or pouring cream.

BONUS POINT
• Chocolate contains theobromines and other 'feel-good' substances that encourage feelings of pleasure and warmth.

OKAY FOR UNDER-ONES?
Not suitable. See pages 16-19 for other ideas.

125 g (4 oz) plain dark chocolate
(minimum of 50% cocoa solids),
broken into small pieces
1 tablespoon water
150 g (5 oz) butter
150 g (5 oz) caster sugar
4 eggs, beaten
1 teaspoon vanilla extract
175 g (6 oz) self-raising flour
25 g (1 oz) cocoa powder
1 teaspoon baking powder
75 ml (3 fl oz) milk or water

• If you don't eat this pudding at once you may find the chocolatey 'puddle' at the bottom disappears, as it is absorbed by the sponge.
• To make individual puddings, bake the mixture in 4 buttered individual ovenproof dishes for 20 minutes only.

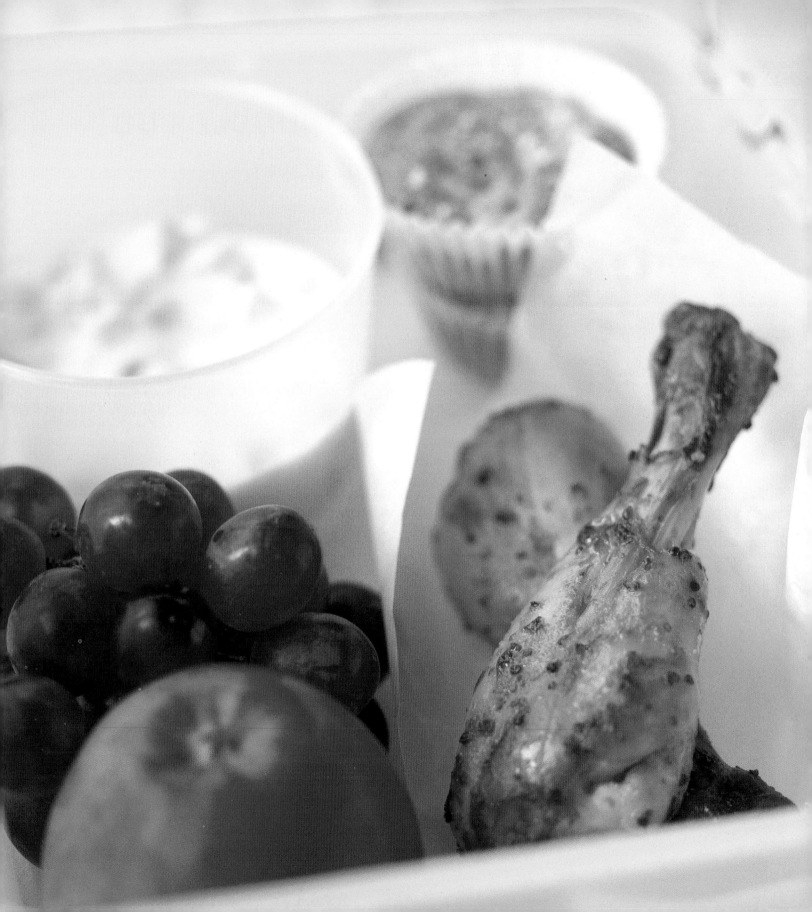

Packed Lunch

There's always something exciting about opening a packed lunch – a sense of expectation, hope and mystery. And it's easy to make sure that what's inside lives up to the promise – all you need is a little forward thought and planning. Remember it's just as important for a packed lunch to be nutritious as it is for any other main meal. A good balance of foods will help your child – or your partner, or you – to be on good form right through the afternoon.

WIZARD DRUMSTICKS

150 ml (¼ pint) Greek yogurt

2 tablespoons redcurrant jelly

1 tablespoon wholegrain mustard

1 garlic clove, crushed

grated rind and juice of ½ lemon

6-8 chicken drumsticks, skinned if preferred

black pepper

Chicken is always a hit, especially when it's baked barbecue-style, as here. On baking, these marinated drumsticks take on a lovely shiny brown colour, inviting you to pick them up and eat. Bake the drumsticks the day before so they are cool the next morning, ready to be packed into the lunch box.

To make the marinade, mix the yogurt, redcurrant jelly, mustard, garlic, lemon rind and juice together in a bowl and season with pepper.

Add the chicken drumsticks to the bowl and, with clean hands, turn them to coat thoroughly with the mixture. Cover and leave to marinate in the refrigerator for at least 30 minutes, preferably several hours.

Turn the chicken and transfer to a roasting tin. Bake in a preheated oven at 190°C (375°F) Gas Mark 5 for 40-45 minutes, basting and turning halfway through cooking, until golden brown and cooked through. Allow to cool.

Wrap the drumsticks in non-stick paper before adding to the lunch box.

BONUS POINT
• Chicken is an excellent source of protein (for growth and repair).

OKAY FOR UNDER-ONES?
To make the marinade milder, use only 1 teaspoon of mustard.

4 months Not suitable. Give mashed potato moistened with milk or water.

5-6 months Blend some chicken with a little milk or water and cooked potato.

6-9 months As above, or finely mince chicken with raita and serve mashed potato separately.

10-12 months Finely chop chicken and raita; serve with mashed potato.

• A small tub of raita for dipping the drumsticks into is the perfect complement: Mix 175 ml (6 fl oz) natural 'bio' yogurt with 10 cm (4 inches) cucumber, chopped.

• Add kitchen paper to the lunch box for cleaning hands afterwards. Individually wrapped moist wipes are ideal if your child can be persuaded to use them.

CHEESY VEGETABLE PASTIES

These mini pasties make tasty snacks or packed lunch fillers, and you can vary the choice of vegetables in the filling to suit your family's tastes – sweetcorn, green beans and courgettes are equally suitable. It's well worth making double the quantity of pasties, so you can freeze half of them in individual bags for other days. *Makes 8*

Pastry:

125 g (4 oz) plain wholemeal flour

125 g (4 oz) plain white flour

150 g (5 oz) unsalted butter, cut into small pieces

2 tablespoons cold water (approximately)

Filling:

3 tablespoons olive, rapeseed (canola) or walnut oil

1 small onion, finely chopped

2 teaspoons plain flour

225 ml (7 fl oz) milk

75 g (3 oz) Cheddar cheese, grated

1 medium carrot, grated

1 small potato, finely diced

125 g (4 oz) broccoli florets, cut into small pieces

50 g (2 oz) frozen peas

beaten egg, to glaze

To make the pastry, put the flours in a food processor, add the butter and process until the mixture resembles breadcrumbs. Add the water and work briefly to a smooth dough, adding a little more water if necessary. Wrap and chill in the refrigerator while preparing the filling.

Heat the oil in a saucepan. Add the onion and fry for 3 minutes. Stir in the flour, then add the milk, cheese, carrot, potato, broccoli and peas. Bring to the boil and cook for 2 minutes, stirring constantly, until the sauce has thickened. Leave to cool.

Divide the dough into 8 portions. Roll out each piece to a 16 cm (6½ inch) round, using a small plate as a guide. Trim the edges and brush with beaten egg. Divide the filling between the pastry rounds, placing it in the centres. Bring the edges of the pastry up over the filling and press together firmly to make pasty shapes. Crimp the edges, using your fingers.

Transfer to a greased baking sheet and brush with beaten egg. Bake in a preheated oven at 200°C (400°F) Gas Mark 6 for about 25 minutes until the pastry is golden. Transfer to a wire rack to cool. Allow to cool completely if the pasties are for a packed lunch.

Serve the pasties warm or cold, with cherry tomatoes or a tomato salad if you like.

BONUS POINTS
• The wholemeal flour in the pastry is a good source of fibre.
• Milk, flour and carrots provide plenty of calcium – essential for growing children, to ensure strong bones and teeth.

OKAY FOR UNDER-ONES?
4-6 months Not suitable. Give some lightly steamed and suitably moistened puréed broccoli, carrot or potato instead, perhaps with a few peas mashed in for babies already used to the other flavours.
6-12 months Blend the food for babies who can't yet cope with lumps. Cut the pastry and broccoli florets up small for older babies.

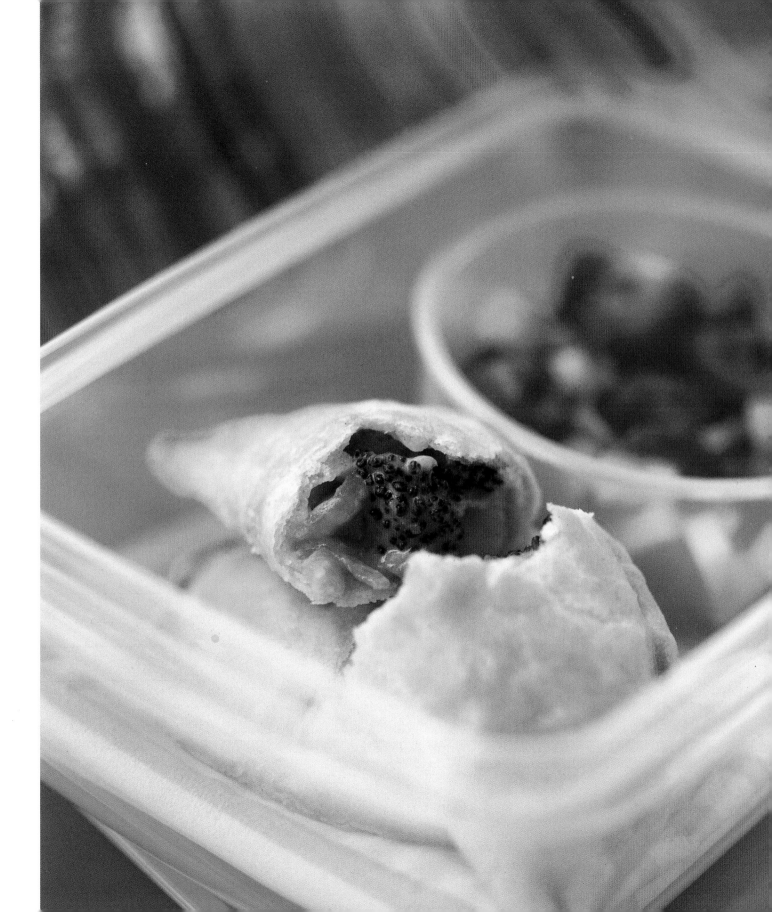

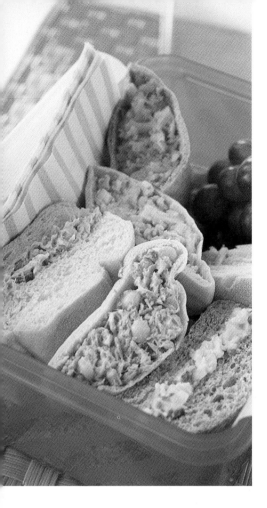

SANDWICHES

Variety is the key to appetizing sandwiches, but remember it isn't just the flavour of the filling that's important, but also its texture and moistness, together with the type of bread, and the sort of spread.

Bread

Vary the type of bread you use for sandwiches. Bread made from white or brown wheat flour doesn't have quite as many nutrients, or as much fibre, as bread made from wholemeal flour – which contains the whole of the grain. So it's a good idea to encourage your family to eat wholemeal bread most of the time. If a child doesn't like wholemeal, try giving them white bread that contains added fibre. Bread made with rye or barley flour, oatmeal, or mixed grain flour is delicious for a change. Pumpernickel is often popular, too.

Breads containing whole seeds or chopped nuts are undoubtedly delicious and nutritionally excellent, but not advisable for children under the age of five, because of the small risk of choking on a seed or piece of nut.

Don't restrict sandwiches to sliced bread. For variety, use rolls, baps, chunks of a French stick, and mini baguettes, too. Pitta bread can also be split and filled. You can also sandwich fillings between wholegrain crackers or rice cakes, for a change.

Spreads

Don't always opt for butter or a similar sort of fat to spread on bread. Use your imagination and choose an original spread that complements the flavour of the filling, and perhaps adds nourishment and zing. A spread between the bread and filling helps to keep sandwiches moist, but it isn't always essential. Some foods can be used either as a spread or a filling, though you would use more as a filling. Here are some ideas:

• Avocado, mashed with 1 teaspoon lemon juice
• Butter, at room temperature, or 'spreadable' (not low-fat for under-fives)
• Cream cheese or curd cheese (full-fat for under-fives)
• Fromage frais (full-fat for under-fives)
• Horseradish sauce (not for under-ones)
• Hummus (see page 138)
• Mayonnaise (avoid low-fat mayonnaise for under-fives)
• Olive oil margarine
• Olive tapenade (not for under-ones)
• Peanut butter (see tip box)

• Peanut butter is popular with many children, but it can cause a serious allergic reaction. Increasingly, schools are requesting that parents don't send children to school with any food containing peanuts, particularly if there is a known child with a peanut allergy. Even a tiny morsel of peanut butter sandwich could set off a potentially fatal reaction if a child has an acute allergy problem. So, do check with your child's school before packing peanut butter sandwiches in their lunch box.

• Put the sandwiches in a little plastic bag to keep them moist for a packed lunch.
• Bread for sandwiches must be very fresh. Small rolls and slices from a cut loaf can taken from the freezer and filled while still frozen – the sandwiches will be thawed in time for lunch.

Fillings

Try the following nutritious ideas (quantities are per sandwich):
• **Beetroot and cream cheese:** Mix 50 g (2 oz) of grated cooked beetroot (not in vinegar) with 1 tablespoon of cream cheese. Stir in ½-1 teaspoon of horseradish sauce if liked.
• **BLT (bacon, lettuce and tomato):** Roughly crumble 2 rashers crisp-grilled back bacon and mix with 2 tablespoons sliced lettuce and 1 sliced tomato.
• **Cheese and olive:** Mix 25 g (1 oz) of grated Edam cheese with 1-2 pitted and chopped green or black olives.
• **Chicken and aubergine:** Lay one slice of roast chicken over 2 roasted or grilled slices of aubergine.
• **Chicken and avocado:** Mash ⅓-½ avocado with 1 teaspoon lemon juice. Chop 2 slices roast chicken and mix with the avocado.
• **Cucumber and sardine:** Mash 1 canned sardine and spread on one of the bread slices. Top with cucumber slices.
• **Egg and cress or celery:** Mash 1 cooled hard-boiled egg with 2 teaspoons mayonnaise. Stir in a little cress or finely chopped celery.
• **Liver sausage and lettuce:** Sandwich the bread with 2-4 slices of liver sausage and lettuce leaves. Low-fat mayonnaise is an ideal spread.
• **Orange cheese and carrot:** Mix 1 finely grated carrot with 25 g (1 oz) of Double Gloucester or Red Leicester cheese. Add a little chutney, if liked.
• **Salmon and lettuce:** Mash 50 g (2 oz) canned salmon with 1 tablespoon of mayonnaise. Sandwich the bread with the salmon and lettuce leaves.
• **Tuna and red pepper:** Mash 50 g (2 oz) canned tuna, then mix with a little finely chopped red pepper. Stir in 1 tablespoon of canned sweetcorn, if liked.

BONUS POINT

• Provided you opt for a nutritious filling, an entire balanced meal can be packed into 1 or 2 sandwiches.

OKAY FOR UNDER-ONES?

Don't give babies sandwiches with bacon, olives, liver sausage, horseradish, peanut butter, chutney or olive tapenade.
4-6 months Not suitable. Give some avocado or banana mashed with milk or water. Babies of 5 months can have some chicken blended with a little water.
6-9 months Cut a sandwich with a soft filling into very small pieces, and soften with milk or water. A harder filling such as chicken must be blended separately. You can also bake a piece of bread and give it to your baby as a rusk.
9-12 months When your baby can chew, give him or her a sandwich with a soft filling to hold. Chicken and other meat is still difficult to chew, so you may need to mince or blend it until around 10 months, and give separately.

IT'S A WRAP!

4-8 flour tortillas

Chicken fajitas filling:

2 tablespoons corn, olive or rapeseed
  (canola) oil

½ teaspoon cayenne pepper

2 teaspoons lemon juice

6 tablespoons Greek yogurt

375 g (12 oz) skinless chicken breast, cut
  into strips

1 onion, chopped

1 garlic clove, crushed

2 carrots, finely sliced

1 green pepper, chopped (optional)

• Soft wraps are delicious filled with
Every Flavour Beans (see page 69) –
plain or spicy. Put a spoonful of
beans to one side of the centre of
each soft wrap, then wrap the
unfilled half over the filling.

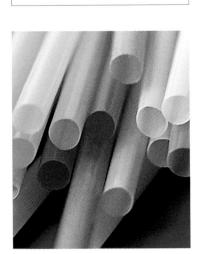

Food wrapped in a parcel always tastes twice as delightful, especially if the wrapping is edible. Flour tortillas (available from most supermarkets); wheat flour 'soft wraps' (from selected supermarkets); and little rice flour pancakes (from large supermarkets, or Chinese food stores) all make perfect wrappings for savoury fillings. Experiment with the following ideas, or your own choice of filling.

For the filling, in a large bowl mix 1 tablespoon of the oil with the cayenne, lemon juice and yogurt. Add the chicken and stir to coat in the mixture. Leave to marinate in a cool place for 30 minutes, if possible.

Heat the remaining oil in a large frying pan. Add the onion, garlic and carrots, and cook gently for 5 minutes, stirring from time to time. Add the marinated chicken and green pepper (if using), and fry gently, stirring occasionally, for 15 minutes, until the chicken is cooked through.

If serving immediately, fill the tortillas at once; otherwise allow the filling to cool before filling. Divide the filling between the flour tortillas, placing it to one side of the centre. Wrap the unfilled half around the filling.

For a lunch box, wrap in non-stick baking paper. Serve with a salad or cherry tomatoes. If serving warm, accompany with a lightly steamed green leafy vegetable, such as spinach, cabbage or Brussels sprouts.

BONUS POINTS
• Wraps are a child-friendly way of parcelling up vegetables and contributing towards the 5 recommended helpings of vegetables and fruits a day.

OKAY FOR UNDER-ONES?
4-6 months Not suitable. Instead, give a little steamed carrot or green leafy vegetable, mashed with milk or water. Babies of 5 months can have some cooked chicken, blended with milk or water and a little steamed carrot.
6-12 months Give some of the chicken filling, blended with a little extra yogurt. Or, when the baby can chew well (probably around 10 months), give some of the flour tortilla wrap and filling, cut up very small. From 9 months babies can have some of the soft wrap with beans cut up small, moistened with a little milk or water if necessary.

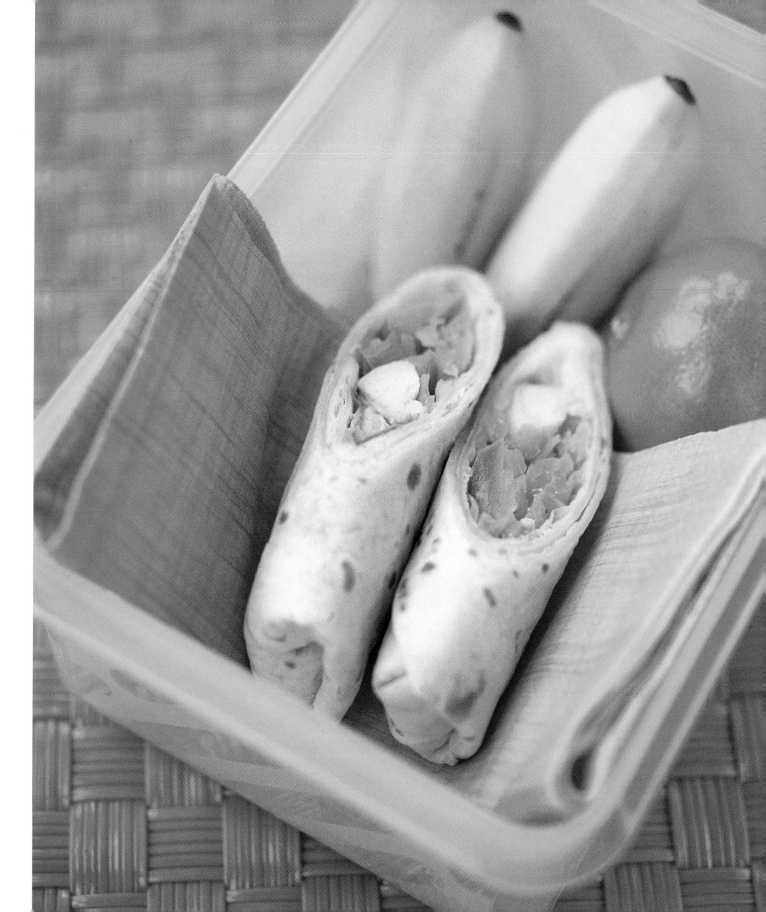

DIPS, 'DUNKERS' & NIBBLES

SUITABLE DUNKERS:

• Strips of pitta bread; Herby Bread Sticks (see page 137); and chunks of French stick (preferably wholemeal)

• Crackers (preferably wholegrain); Cheese Straws (see page 135); and Vegetable Crisps (see page 136)

• Sticks of celery, carrot, cucumber or red pepper; raw cauliflower florets; canned baby sweetcorn

• Romaine, chicory or other crisp salad leaves

• Apple or pear quarters, and chunks of banana (all dipped in lemon juice to prevent browning)

• Strawberries; cherry tomatoes

• Chicken drumsticks (see page 109); strips of grilled chicken breast

• Sticks of Cheddar, Edam or other 'hard' cheese

OTHER IDEAS FOR NIBBLES:

• Whole banana, pear, apple, plums, blueberries, seedless grapes or strawberries

• Large chunks of mango or melon (dipped in lemon juice)

• Rings of fresh pineapple (or pineapple canned in natural juice)

• Ready-to-eat dried apricots and prunes; raisins

• Hard-boiled egg wedges

• Olives (pitted for under-fives)

A packed lunch box is a perfect vehicle for healthy 'nibbles'. Mix and match them along with any bigger items, like sandwiches, to provide an enjoyable, well balanced meal. A little tub of fresh dip, together with foods to eat it with, makes a welcome addition to any lunch box. Dips and 'dunkers' are also good party food and snacks.

Dips should be tasty, moreish, and thick enough to be scooped with 'dunkers'. Cover dips closely with clingfilm if you make them ahead of time, or they may darken and dry on the surface. Pack nibbles, dunkers and dips separately in small plastic tubs for inclusion in lunch boxes. Try the following ideas:

Cream cheese and pineapple dip: Mix 125 g (4 oz) cream cheese with 1 tablespoon mayonnaise and 2 peeled, cored and chopped rings of fresh pineapple (or canned in natural juice). Add 25 g (1 oz) of diced ham if you like.
Hummus: Make your own, if possible (see page 138).
Tuna dip: Blend ½ small onion, 175 g (6 oz) tuna canned in oil, 1 tablespoon fromage frais or mayonnaise, and 1 tablespoon chopped fresh parsley.
Yogurt and date dip: Mix 175 ml (6 fl oz) thick creamy yogurt with 50 g (2 oz) chopped stoned dates.

OKAY FOR UNDER-ONES?

Don't give them crackers, baby sweetcorn, ham, or the Yogurt and date dip.
4-6 months Not suitable. Instead, give lightly steamed carrots, cauliflower or broccoli, blended or mashed with a little cooking water or milk. Or give banana or ripe pear, mashed with milk or water. Or, from 5 months, give some chicken blended with some steamed vegetables and a little water.
6-9 months Use any of the suggestions for 4-6 months, gradually making the food less smooth. Chicken needs blending with a little water, or mincing. You can also give mashed blueberries, strawberries, seedless grapes and mango.
9-12 months Once your baby can chew, cut the food up small, and include a little cucumber. Offer cut up pineapple, or grated cheese. Chicken needs chopping and blending with a little water and steamed vegetable, or mincing, until a child is around 10 months. Babies old enough to hold pieces of bread, raw carrot, fruit or cheese will enjoy sucking them or, when old enough, biting off bits to chew. Either cut up the 'dunkers', or let an older baby use them to scoop up some dip from their plate or bowl.

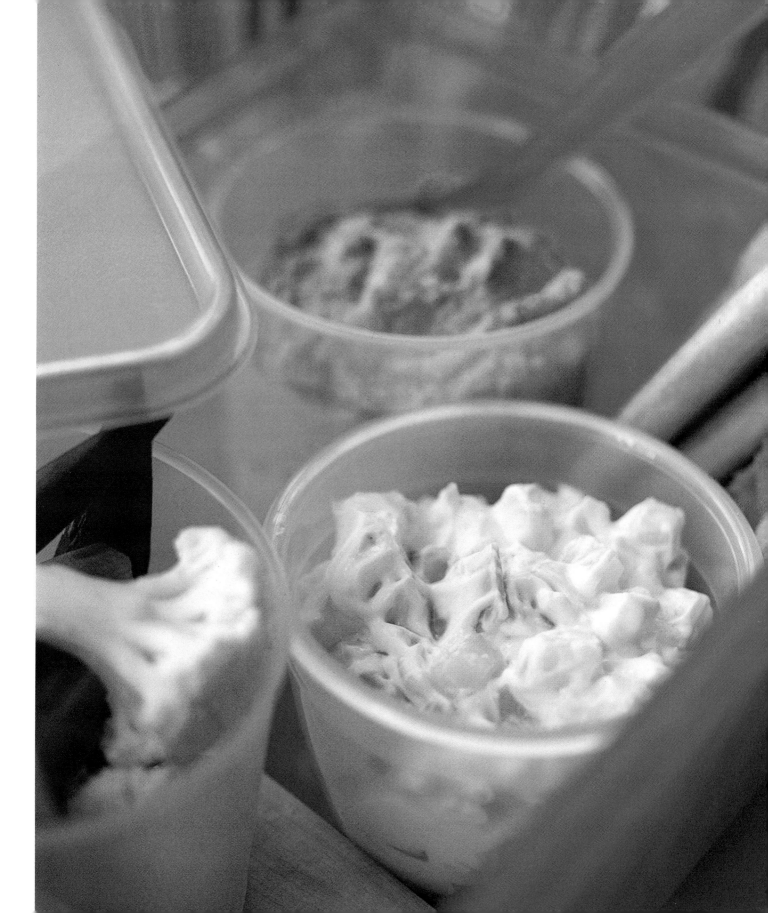

FRUIT & RICE SALAD

50 g (2 oz) split red lentils

200 g (7 oz) long-grain rice

2 mandarins, clementines or small
    oranges

2 kiwi fruit

6 tablespoons fresh orange juice

2 tablespoons clear honey (optional)

• Always slip a pre-frozen freezer pack into your child's lunch box, to ensure the contents remain fresh. On a hot day it is essential, but during the winter you may find that lunch boxes are kept near a radiator during the morning.

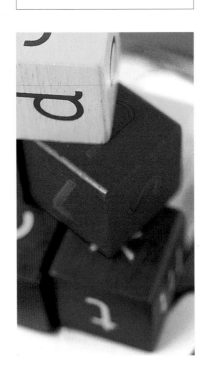

You probably haven't thought of mixing lentils with fruit before. Yet the combination – along with rice – is really excellent. The orangey-red of the lentils echoes the colour of the mandarins and they both complement the green of the kiwis to make a pretty salad. Prepare it the night before, ready to put into a tub for a packed lunch next day.

Put the lentils in a small pan, cover with boiling water and cook for about 10 minutes until the lentils are tender but retaining their shape. Drain and rinse under cold running water.

Meanwhile, cook the rice in a separate pan until tender. Drain and rinse under cold running water; drain well.

Cut the skins from the oranges, removing the pith as well as the peel, then chop the flesh. Peel and chop the kiwi fruit. Blend the orange juice with the honey (if using). Combine all of the ingredients in a bowl, cover and chill until required.

Serve with cold meat, such as chicken or turkey; or fish, especially salmon and tuna.

BONUS POINTS
• There is plenty of vitamin C in this salad from the kiwi, citrus fruit and orange juice.
• The lentils provide long-lasting energy and a little protein.

OKAY FOR UNDER-ONES?
Omit the honey for under-ones; the oranges should provide enough natural sweetness.

4-6 months Not suitable, because although each ingredient (apart from honey) can be offered to young babies, the combination of so many foods would be too much. Instead, give some mashed kiwi fruit, or rice pudding (see page 106), or, for babies who have already tried both, a combination of the two.

6-12 months Blend the food until your baby is able to cope with pieces, then cut up small.

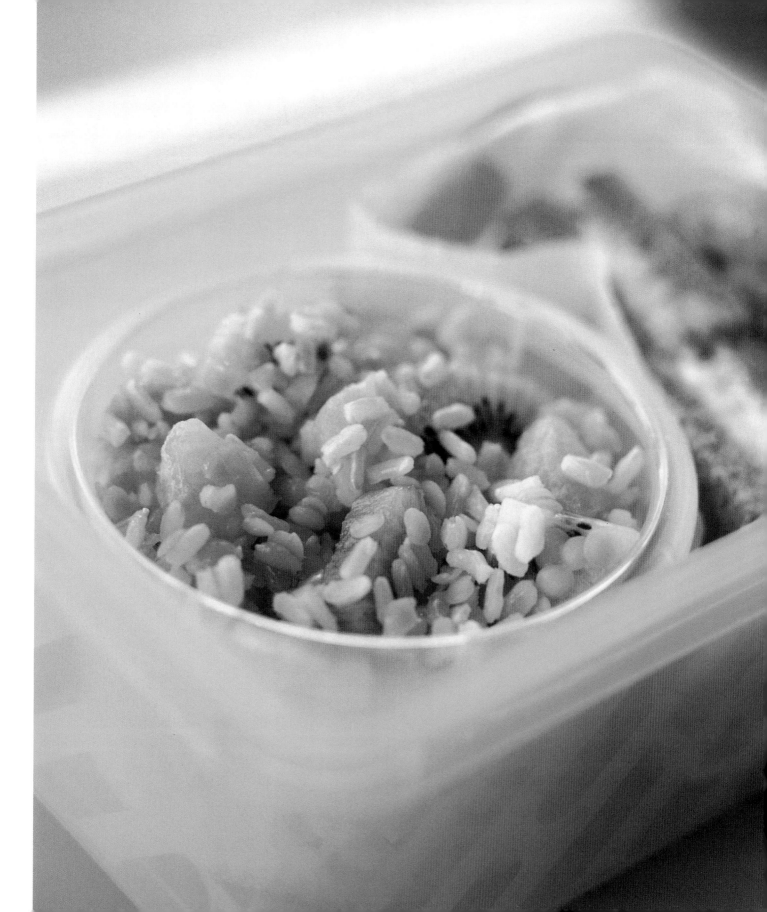

COUSCOUS SALAD

This unusual salad with its sweet-savoury flavours keeps well in the refrigerator for a couple of days, ready and waiting to fill a lunch box or make a healthy snack.

200 g (7 oz) couscous

250 ml (8 fl oz) hot fresh vegetable stock (see page 51)

2 red-skinned dessert apples, cored and diced

125 g (4 oz) Cheddar cheese, diced

75 g (3 oz) sultanas

8 tablespoons apple juice

2 tablespoons chopped flat leaf parsley (optional)

Put the couscous in a bowl and pour on the hot stock. Cover and leave for 15 minutes until the stock is completely absorbed. Turn the couscous into a cold bowl and fluff up the grains with a fork to separate. Leave to cool.

Add the diced apples, cheese, sultanas, apple juice and parsley (if using), and toss together until evenly combined. Cover and chill until required.

Serve with hot or cold meat or fish; or roasted vegetables, such as aubergine slices.

BONUS POINT
• The apple and sultanas together form one of the 5 daily recommended portions of fruit and vegetables.

OKAY FOR UNDER-ONES?
4-6 months Not suitable. Give stewed eating apple, sweetened with a little apple juice or milk if necessary. Or mash some aubergine flesh with a little stock.

6-12 months Blend or thoroughly mash to break up the apple and sultanas until your baby is old enough – perhaps at 8 or 9 months – to chew them.

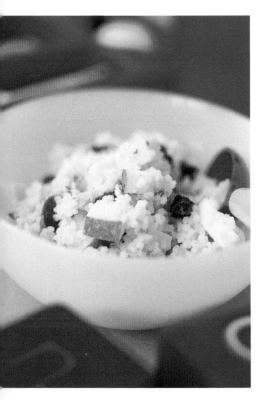

• Vary this salad by including other fruits, such as grapes, chopped dried apricots or prunes.
• As for cheese, try Edam, Gruyère or mozzarella instead of Cheddar.

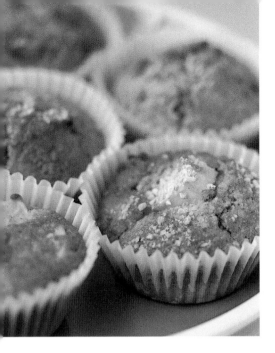

OAT & APPLE MUFFINS

Muffins are some of the easiest cakes to make and they are perfect for lunch-box fillers. They're also very good served warm for breakfast – simply pop into the microwave for about 20 seconds. Muffins are best eaten fresh within 24 hours of baking, or frozen on the day they are made. *Makes 12*

125 g (4 oz) plain white flour

125 g (4 oz) wholemeal plain flour

1 tablespoon baking powder

50 g (2 oz) medium oatmeal

50 g (2 oz) light muscovado sugar

3 small dessert apples, peeled, cored and diced

50 g (2 oz) sultanas or raisins

50 g (2 oz) unsalted butter, melted and cooled slightly

150 ml (¼ pint) yogurt

150 ml (¼ pint) milk

1 egg

5 tablespoons clear honey (see tip box)

a little extra oatmeal, for dusting

• If you intend to give muffins to under-ones, omit the honey and use double the quantity of sugar instead.

• If preferred make smaller muffins in ordinary 'fairy cake' sized paper cakes. The mixture will make about 24 in two bun tin trays. Reduce the cooking time to 15-18 minutes.

Line a 12-hole muffin tray or deep bun tin with paper muffin cases. Mix the flours, baking powder, oatmeal and sugar in a bowl. Stir in the chopped apples and sultanas or raisins.

In another bowl, beat together the butter, yogurt, milk, egg and honey. Add this mixture to the dry ingredients and stir quickly and briefly, until just incorporated; do not over-mix.

Divide the mixture between the paper cases and sprinkle with a little extra oatmeal. Bake in a preheated oven at 200°C (400°F) Gas Mark 6 for 18-20 minutes until just firm to the touch. Transfer to a wire rack to cool.

Pop the cold muffins into a lunch box, or serve warm with stewed apple or plums; or low-sugar plum jam.

BONUS POINT
• Oatmeal is a 'low-GI food' (see Tiredness, page 31); this means it provides long-lasting energy that will help keep your child going without flagging during the morning.

OKAY FOR UNDER-ONES?
Ideally it's better not to give under-ones food containing added sugar.
4-9 months Not suitable. Instead, give some stewed eating apple.
9-12 months The occasional muffin – no more than one a week – won't hurt an older baby, provided teeth and gums are cleaned soon after. However, it's wise to use the extra sugar instead of honey (see tip box), as honey carries a very small risk of potentially problematic food poisoning for under-ones.

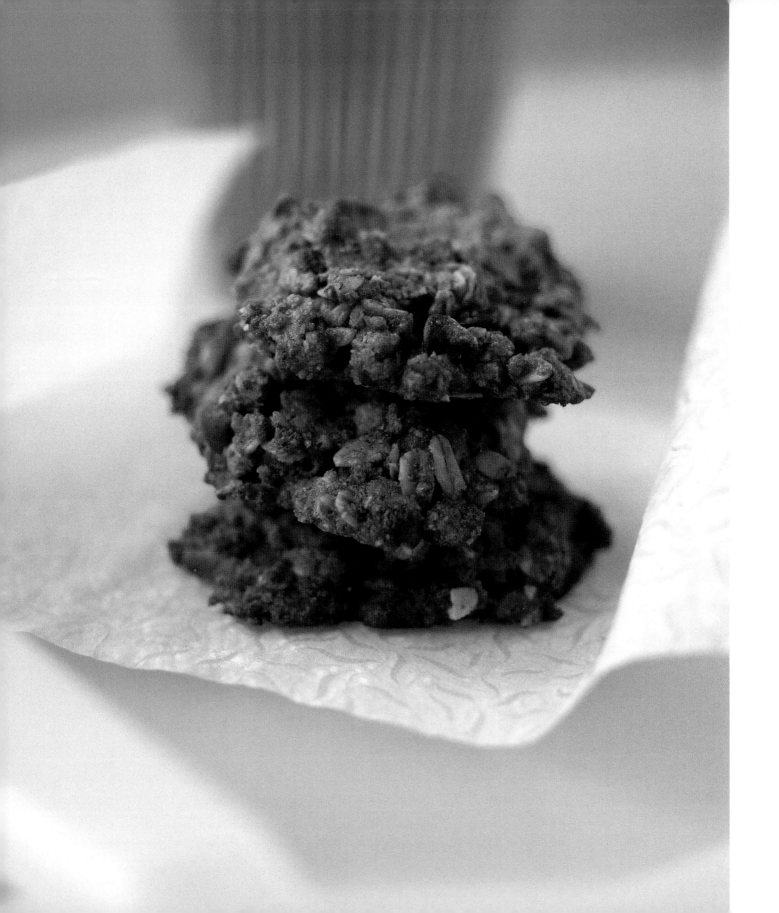

Cakes & Bakes

Fill your kitchen with the wonderful aromas of home-baked bread, cakes and cookies and it will act like a magnet drawing your family in for a welcome treat. Shop-bought baked goods are usually of a reasonable quality, but they generally contain additives and are almost always more expensive. Home baking enables you to determine exactly what your family are eating, saves you money, and gives more delicious results.

CHOCOLATE CRUMBLES

These delectable cookies are laden with chocolate and therefore need little extra sugar. They are also packed with oats and wholemeal flour, which makes them a good source of lasting energy. *Makes 14-16*

125 g (4 oz) plain wholemeal flour

1 teaspoon baking powder

125 g (4 oz) porridge oats

125 g (4 oz) unsalted butter, melted and cooled slightly

40 g (1½ oz) light muscovado sugar

1 egg, beaten

150 g (5 oz) good quality plain, milk or white chocolate, in small pieces

• For an extra chocolatey flavour, use dark chocolate that contains a minimum of 70% cocoa solids.

• Butter and chocolate are high in saturated fat, so discourage older children from pigging out on these cookies; if they do, cut down on the fat – and saturated fat in particular – they have for the rest of the day.

Mix the flour, baking powder and oats together in a bowl. Add the butter, sugar, egg and chocolate and beat until evenly combined.

Take dessertspoonfuls of the mixture and pat roughly into cakes. Place slightly apart on a greased large baking sheet. Bake in a preheated oven at 200°C (400°F) Gas Mark 6 for about 15 minutes until slightly risen and lightly coloured. Leave on the baking sheet for 2 minutes, then cool on a wire rack.

Store in an airtight container for up to 4 days. Serve as a snack, or with some fresh raspberries or strawberries and fromage frais as a dessert.

BONUS POINTS
• The cocoa solids in chocolate – especially the dark 70% cocoa-solid variety – provide vitamin B which is good for nerves, and antioxidants that help keep the arteries healthy in young and old alike.
• Wholemeal flour contains more fibre and vitamin B than white flour, and the oats are an added bonus.

OKAY FOR UNDER-ONES?
4-9 months Not suitable. See pages 16-19 for other alternatives.
9-12 months It's best not to give under-ones food with added sugar, and that includes chocolate. However, the occasional cookie – perhaps once a week – won't hurt an older baby, provided the teeth and gums are cleaned afterwards.

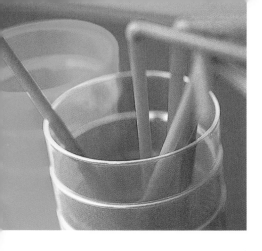

APRICOT PUFFED RICE BARS

These make a good teatime treat, can be popped into lunch boxes, and are fine as an after-supper filler for children too. They are also much cheaper than their ready-made equivalents. *Makes 12-16*

25 g (1 oz) unsalted butter, cut into small pieces

125 g (4 oz) mini marshmallows, halved, or whole marshmallows, quartered

2 tablespoons golden syrup

75 g (3 oz) dried apricots, peaches or mangoes, finely chopped

125 g (4 oz) puffed rice breakfast cereal (such as Rice Krispies)

• Both pink and white marsh-mallows can be used. As these are rich in refined carbohydrate, check that your family has plenty of fibre-rich foods during the rest of the day.

Line a 25 x 18 cm (10 x 7 inch) Swiss roll tin with non-stick baking paper, or spray with vegetable oil cooking spray.

Melt the butter, marshmallows and golden syrup together in a large saucepan over a low heat until smooth, stirring frequently. Take off the heat and stir in the apricots and puffed rice cereal to coat thoroughly.

Spoon the mixture into the prepared tin and smooth the surface. Allow to cool and firm up for at least 1 hour. Cut into bars to serve.

BONUS POINTS
• Puffed rice is enriched with B vitamins – for growth, energy and healthy nerves.
• Apricots, peaches and mangoes are rich in beta-carotene, a plant pigment that helps protect cells from damage.

OKAY FOR UNDER-ONES?
4-6 months Not suitable. Alternatives for a mid-morning or teatime snack include mashed ripe dessert pear moistened with a little milk or apple juice if necessary, or stewed eating apple.
6-12 months Not suitable. Alternative snacks as above or, for babies who can chew, offer baked bread rusks, crumpet fingers or toast soldiers.

STRAWBERRY RING COOKIES

A blend of ground almonds and ground rice give these mildly spiced, wheat-free cookies a lovely moist, crumbly texture, and the small dollop of jam in the middle adds a little sweetness. *Makes 12*

200 g (7 oz) ground almonds

50 g (2 oz) ground rice

1 teaspoon ground mixed spice (optional)

5 tablespoons clear honey

50 g (2 oz) unsalted butter

1 egg yolk

2 teaspoons vanilla extract

3 tablespoons low-sugar strawberry or
    raspberry jam

Mix the ground almonds, rice and spice (if using) together in a bowl.

Put the honey and butter in a small pan and heat gently until the butter is melted. Pour the mixture into the bowl. Add the egg yolk and vanilla extract and mix until evenly combined. Roll dessertspoonfuls of the mixture into balls. Place on a greased large baking sheet and flatten slightly. Press a deep hole into the centre of each with the finger.

Spoon about a teaspoonful of the jam into each biscuit. Bake in a preheated oven at 180°C (350°F) Gas Mark 4 for 15-20 minutes until pale golden. Leave on the baking sheet for 2 minutes, then transfer to a wire rack to cool. Store in an airtight container for up to 2 days. Serve the cookies on their own, or with fresh sliced strawberries.

BONUS POINTS
• Ground almonds are a good source of magnesium, iron and zinc, and provide more calcium than any other nuts. Eating the cookies with vitamin C-rich strawberries aids the absorption of these minerals.

OKAY FOR UNDER-ONES?
These are not recommended. Instead, give mashed strawberries, or an alternative snack (see left for suggestions).

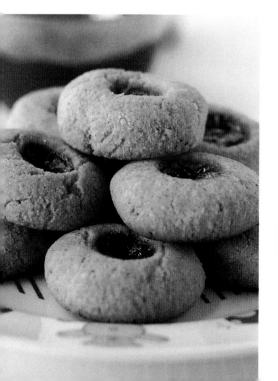

• Avoid overfilling these cookies with jam, or it may boil out during baking.
• Don't let enthusiastic little fingers pick up a cookie before it has properly cooled, as jam retains heat longer than you might think.

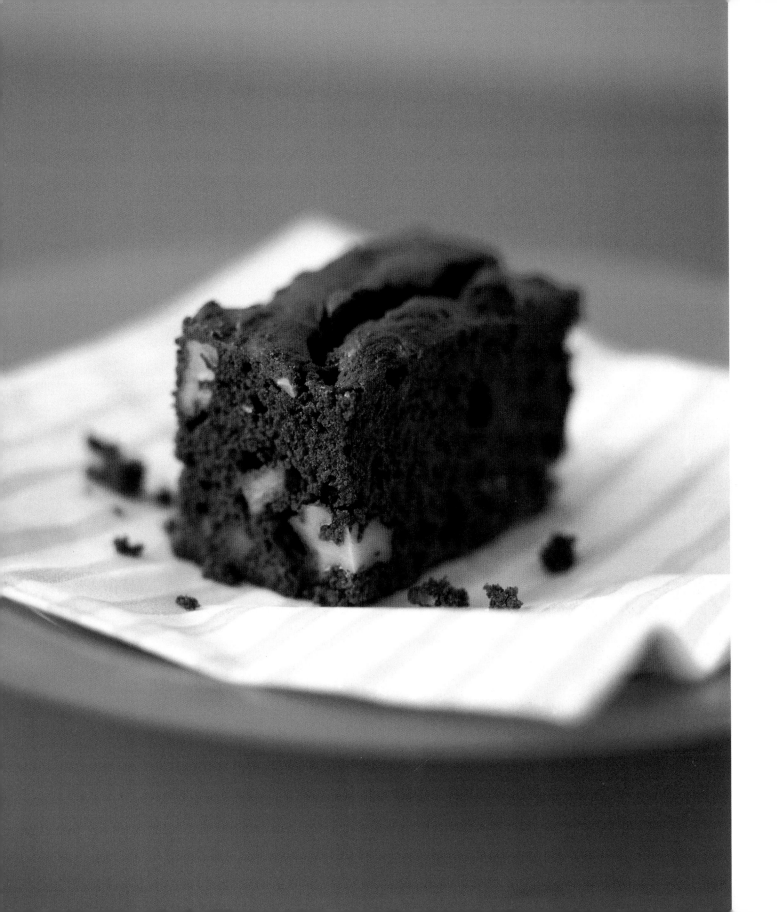

BROWNIES

Luscious chocolate brownies are an irresistible treat at any time of the day. Served with Greek yogurt, they also make a delicious dessert. Most children like plain brownies, without walnuts or pecans, though melt-in-the-mouth chunks of creamy white chocolate are a popular addition (see tip box). Brownies freeze well, but unless you make double the quantity your family will probably devour them before they reach the freezer. *Makes 20*

50 g (2 oz) butter

2 tablespoons rapeseed (canola) or walnut oil

2 eggs, beaten

125 g (4 oz) muscovado sugar

1 teaspoon vanilla extract

125 g (4 oz) self-raising flour

40 g (1½ oz) cocoa powder

50 g (2 oz) dried cherries, chopped (optional)

50 g (2 oz) ground hazelnuts (optional)

Line a 20 cm (8 inch) square cake tin with non-stick baking paper.

Melt the butter in a large pan over a low heat. Remove from the heat and mix in the oil, eggs, sugar and vanilla extract. Then stir in the flour and cocoa powder, followed by the dried cherries and ground hazelnuts (if using).

Bake in a preheated oven at 180°C (350°F) Gas Mark 4 for 30 minutes. Remove from the oven, leave to stand for 10 minutes, then cut into squares. Allow the brownies to cool completely before removing from the tin.

Serve brownies on their own, or with creamy natural yogurt as a dessert.

BONUS POINTS
• Cocoa powder, made from crushed cocoa beans, is rich in antioxidant flavonoids that help prevent cells from damage.
• Nuts contain the essential fatty acids needed for the healthy production of hormones and natural anti-inflammatory substances.
• The aroma of chocolate or cocoa during baking boosts 'feel-good' hormones called endorphins, which is rewarding in itself but also boosts immunity.

OKAY FOR UNDER-ONES?
Not suitable, because self-raising flour contains sodium.
4-9 months Instead, give mashed stewed apricot or eating apple, or mashed raw pitted cherries, ripe peach or pear, moistened if necessary with a little apple juice.
9-12 months Offer one of the above alternatives or, for older babies who can chew, give baked bread rusks, toast soldiers or crumpet fingers.

• For a special treat, add 75 g (3 oz) of white chocolate, roughly cut into 1 cm (½ inch) chunks, omitting the cherries.
• You can buy ready-ground hazelnuts in many supermarkets, but for optimum flavour grind your own in an electric blender.
• Brownies will keep fresh for a couple of days in an airtight tin, but they are best either eaten or frozen on the day they are made.

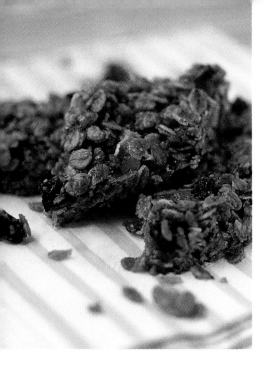

FLAPJACKS

Flapjacks are always popular and this version with its hint of ginger and moist, chewy dried fruit is especially good. You can omit the ginger if you like, though it does give a warm, mildly spicy flavour. *Makes 20*

50 g (2 oz) butter

75 g (3 oz) muscovado sugar

1 teaspoon powdered ginger (optional)

4 tablespoons rapeseed (canola) oil

250 g (8 oz) rolled oats

25 g (1 oz) sultanas

50 g (2 oz) chopped dried apricots, papaya, pears or peaches (or a mixture)

• Flapjacks keep well in an airtight tin, or they can be frozen. Pack in twos or threes in small plastic freezer bags, so you can easily take out a few at a time.

Line a 30 x 20 cm (12 x 8 inch) Swiss roll tin with non-stick baking paper. Put the butter and sugar in a large saucepan and heat gently until melted, then stir in the ginger (if using) and oil. Add the oats, sultanas and fruit, and stir to mix.

Spoon the mixture into the prepared tin, level the surface and press down gently. Bake in a preheated oven at 180°C (350°F) Gas Mark 4 for 30 minutes. Leave in the tin for 10 minutes, then cut into slices. Leave until cold before removing from the tin.

Serve flapjacks on their own, or with stewed apple or plums as a dessert.

BONUS POINTS
• Oats and dried fruit are rich in fibre, and oats are especially rich in soluble fibre – the sort that helps keep blood-sugar level steady and energy from flagging.
• Oats are also rich in B vitamins, which are essential for many tasks – especially releasing energy from food.

OKAY FOR UNDER-ONES?
Not suitable.

4-9 months Instead, give mashed stewed apricot or eating apple, or mashed banana, ripe peach or pear, moistened if necessary with a little apple juice.

9-12 months Offer one of the above alternatives or, for older babies who can chew, give baked bread rusks, toast soldiers or crumpet fingers.

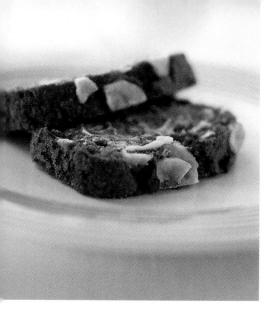

BANANA TEABREAD

This moist, fragrant teabread is perfect for a mid-morning break, packed lunch or picnic treat, and at teatime. Using muscovado sugar, wholemeal flour and rapeseed (canola) oil – instead of the usual white sugar, flour and butter – makes a healthier teabread. *Makes 10-12 slices*

200 g (7 oz) self-raising wholemeal flour

1 teaspoon bicarbonate of soda

½ teaspoon ground mixed spice

75 g (3 oz) muscovado sugar

2 bananas

4 tablespoons rapeseed (canola) or sunflower oil

2 eggs, beaten

4 tablespoons semi-skimmed milk or low-fat yogurt

2 teaspoons vanilla extract

40 g (1½ oz) dried banana chips, chopped

2 tablespoons clear honey, warmed (optional)

Line a 23 x 12 cm (9 x 5 inch) loaf tin with non-stick baking paper, or spray with vegetable oil cooking spray.

Combine the flour, bicarbonate of soda, mixed spice and sugar in a large bowl and make a well in the centre. Mash the bananas and add to the well with the oil, eggs, milk or yogurt, and vanilla extract; stir well. Put the mixture in the prepared loaf tin and smooth the top. Sprinkle with dried banana chips.

Bake in a preheated oven at 180°C (350°F) Gas Mark 4 for 45-50 minutes, or until the loaf is well risen, firm to the touch, and a skewer inserted into the middle comes out clean. On removing from the oven, brush with warm honey to glaze (if desired). Allow to cool.

BONUS POINT
• Bananas provide an excellent, rapidly absorbed source of energy for physically active children and adults.

OKAY FOR UNDER-ONES?
Not suitable, because self-raising flour and bicarbonate of soda contain sodium.
4-9 months Instead, give mashed stewed apricot or eating apple, or mashed banana, ripe peach or pear, moistened if necessary with a little apple juice.
9-12 months Offer one of the above alternatives or, for older babies who can chew, give baked bread rusks, toast soldiers or crumpet fingers.

• Mash the bananas only just before incorporating them into the mixture, otherwise the flesh will turn black as it is oxidised by the air.

CARROT CAKES

One way of ensuring that your children eat enough vegetables and fruit is to incorporate them into as many recipes as you can. Grated carrots and rapeseed (canola) oil make these little cakes deliciously moist. Top them with a cream cheese frosting for extra appeal. *Makes 10*

175 g (6 oz) self-raising wholemeal flour

125 g (4 oz) muscovado sugar

2 teaspoons baking powder

1 teaspoon ground cinnamon

pinch of ground nutmeg

3 eggs, beaten

150 ml (¼ pint) rapeseed (canola) or sunflower oil

1 teaspoon vanilla extract

250 g (8 oz) peeled carrots, grated

Frosting (optional):

75 g (3 oz) low-fat cream cheese

1 teaspoon vanilla extract

50 g (2 oz) icing sugar

To decorate (optional):

small pieces of dried apricot

mint sprigs

• For adults and over-fives, vary these moist cakes by including 100 g (3½ oz) chopped walnuts or pecans. Add them to the mixture with the carrots.

Put the flour, sugar, baking powder, cinnamon and nutmeg into a large bowl, stir to mix, then make a well in the centre. Stir in the eggs, oil, vanilla extract and carrots.

Line 10 sections of a 12-hole muffin tray with paper cases, and spoon the mixture into the cases. Bake in a preheated oven at 180°C (350°F) Gas Mark 4 for 25-30 minutes, until well risen and golden brown. Cool on a wire rack.

To make the frosting (if required), mix the ingredients together in a bowl until smooth. Swirl a teaspoonful of frosting on top of each cake and decorate with pieces of dried apricot and mint sprigs.

Serve these cakes on their own, or as a dessert with low-fat crème fraîche or Greek yogurt.

BONUS POINTS

• Carrots are rich in the orange antioxidant plant pigment, beta-carotene; this helps protect cells from damage, and is particularly useful for protecting the eyes, skin and digestive tract.

• Rapeseed (canola) oil is an excellent replacement for butter in cakes, and provides no saturated fat.

• Both walnuts and pecans provide omega-3 fats, which promote a healthy balance of hormones and help prevent inflammation.

OKAY FOR UNDER-ONES?

These aren't suitable because they contain sugar and sodium (in the baking powder and self-raising flour).

4-9 months Offer an alternative snack, such as mashed or chopped ripe pear moistened if necessary with a little apple juice, or stewed eating apple. (See also pages 16-19.)

9-12 months Give chopped ripe pear or, for older babies who can chew, baked bread rusks, toast soldiers or crumpet fingers.

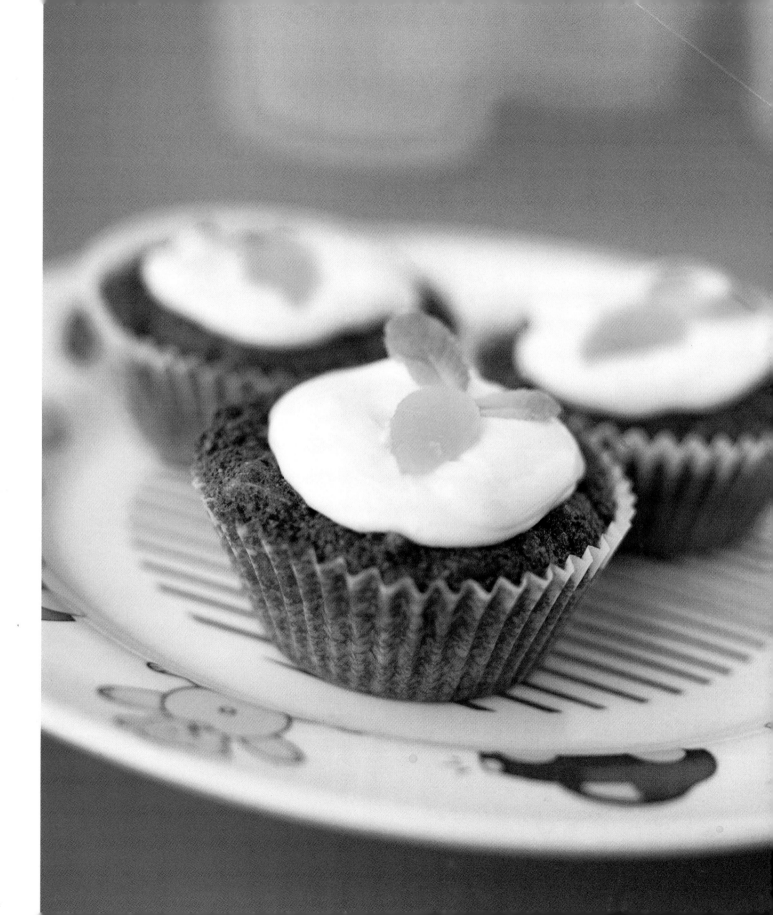

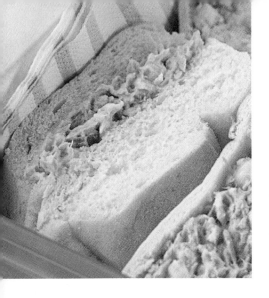

BREAD

Making bread is easy, so if you've never done it before, why not have a go with this recipe. The yeasty fragrance as the bread bakes is wonderful. Most children love to knead dough and make a small loaf of their own. Vary the taste and appearance by adding flavourings (such as herbs, olives or seeds), or by shaping the dough into plaits, rolls or a round loaf.

375 g (12 oz) strong white bread flour

375 g (12 oz) stoneground wholemeal flour

4 teaspoons (two 7 g sachets) easy-blend active dried yeast

50 mg (½ tablet) vitamin C (ascorbic acid), crushed (see tip box)

2 teaspoons sugar

1 tablespoon sunflower or corn oil

450 ml (¾ pint) warm water (see tip box)

• Vitamin C is used to speed the rising process; without it the dough would take about 1½ hours to rise. To crush the ½ tablet, put it in a teaspoon and press the bowl of another teaspoon on top.

• Get the water to just the right temperature by adding 600 ml (1 pint) of cold water to 300 ml (½ pint) boiling water.

• When you knead, repeatedly pull and stretch the dough, as well as kneading it with your knuckles. Kneading is quite hard work and as such it's a form of aerobic exercise!

Lightly oil two 450 g (1 lb) loaf tins, or a large baking sheets if making a round loaf, or bread rolls.

Set aside ½ cupful of the white flour. Put the rest of the flours into a large bowl and make a well in the centre. Add the yeast, vitamin C, sugar, oil and water and mix to a soft dough. Flour the work surface and your hands with the reserved flour, shaking any remaining flour over the dough. Knead the dough on the floured surface for 10 minutes.

Shape the dough into two oblongs, then press into the loaf tins; or shape into one round loaf, or individual rolls and place on the baking sheets, spacing apart to allow room for rising.

Cover with a clean damp tea towel and leave to rise in a warm place for about 30 minutes, or a little longer. Bake in a preheated oven at 230°C (450°F) Gas Mark 8 for 15 minutes, then reduce the setting to 180°C (350°F) Gas Mark 4 and bake loaves for a further 20-25 minutes; or rolls for a further 10-15 minutes. A loaf is cooked when it sounds hollow if tapped firmly on the base. Cool on a wire rack.

Serve with cheese or soup; or use for sandwiches (see pages 112-3), or bruschettas (see pages 60-1); or thinly spread with butter and honey, low-sugar jam, or Marmite.

BONUS POINTS
• Wholemeal flour provides magnesium, zinc, vitamin B6, vitamin E and fibre. It's a better source of nutrients than white flour.

OKAY FOR UNDER-ONES?
Olive and sunflower bread are not suitable for babies. Don't give them honey or Marmite either.

4-6 months Not suitable, because wheat flour contains gluten.

6-9 months Blend bread with a little milk or water; once your baby can cope with lumps, cut it up small and soften by soaking in a little milk or water.

9-12 months Either cut up small, or give your baby some bread to hold.

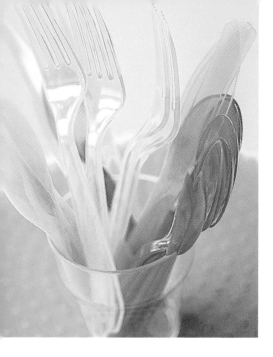

CORNBREAD

Both children and adults love this yellowish cake-like bread. It is excellent hot or cold, can be eaten at once or reheated the next day; it also freezes well. Yellow cornmeal gives the bread a lovely golden colour and pleasant texture; white cornmeal can also be used. Cornflour is altogether different and unsuitable for this recipe.

175 g (6 oz) plain flour

275 g (9 oz) fine yellow cornmeal or polenta flour

2 teaspoons baking powder (optional, see tip box)

pinch of salt (optional)

25 g (1 oz) caster or granulated sugar

100 g (3½ oz) butter, melted

4 eggs, beaten

200 ml (7 fl oz) milk

50 ml (2 fl oz) single cream

• For under-ones you will need to omit the baking powder. As a consequence, the cornbread will have a closer, less spongy texture, but it will still taste good.
• For individual cornbreads, bake the mixture in muffin tins; allow 15-20 minutes in the oven.
• For a flavoured cornbread, add 1 tablespoon of chopped fresh sage and 4 crumbled crisp-grilled rashers of streaky bacon.

Generously butter a 20 cm (8 inch) square baking dish. Put the flour, cornmeal, baking powder, salt and sugar into a bowl, stir to mix and make a well in the centre. Pour in the melted butter, eggs, milk and cream, and mix well until smooth. Shape roughly into a square, a little smaller than the dish.

Warm the dish in the oven preheated to 200°C (400°F) Gas Mark 6 for 5 minutes. Put the cornbread mixture into the dish and bake for 25-30 minutes, or until a skewer inserted into the centre comes out clean. Leave in the tin for 5 minutes, then transfer to a wire rack. Serve warm, cut into squares or slices.

Serve with grilled tomatoes, lean bacon or good quality sausages; or low-sugar cherry jam.

BONUS POINTS
• The mixture of polenta, flour, eggs and milk offers a good balance of nutrients, including fibre (which helps keep the arteries, digestive system and oestrogen-level healthy), protein (for growth and repair of tissues), zinc (especially good for skin, hair, nails and fertility) and vitamins A, B, D and E.
• If you serve cornbread with tomatoes, fry them in a teaspoon of butter or oil to release more lycopene, a useful antioxidant that helps keep cells healthy.

OKAY FOR UNDER-ONES?
Omit the salt and baking powder. Don't serve with bacon or sausages. Although under-ones are better off eating food without added sugar, this cornbread is fine to have occasionally because the amount of sugar is so small. However, it's important to clean your baby's teeth and gums well afterwards.

4-6 months Not suitable. See pages 16-19 for first food ideas.

6-9 months Crumble some cornbread and soften with a little milk or water.

9-12 months Either crumble some cornbread on to a plate, or give your baby a small piece to hold.

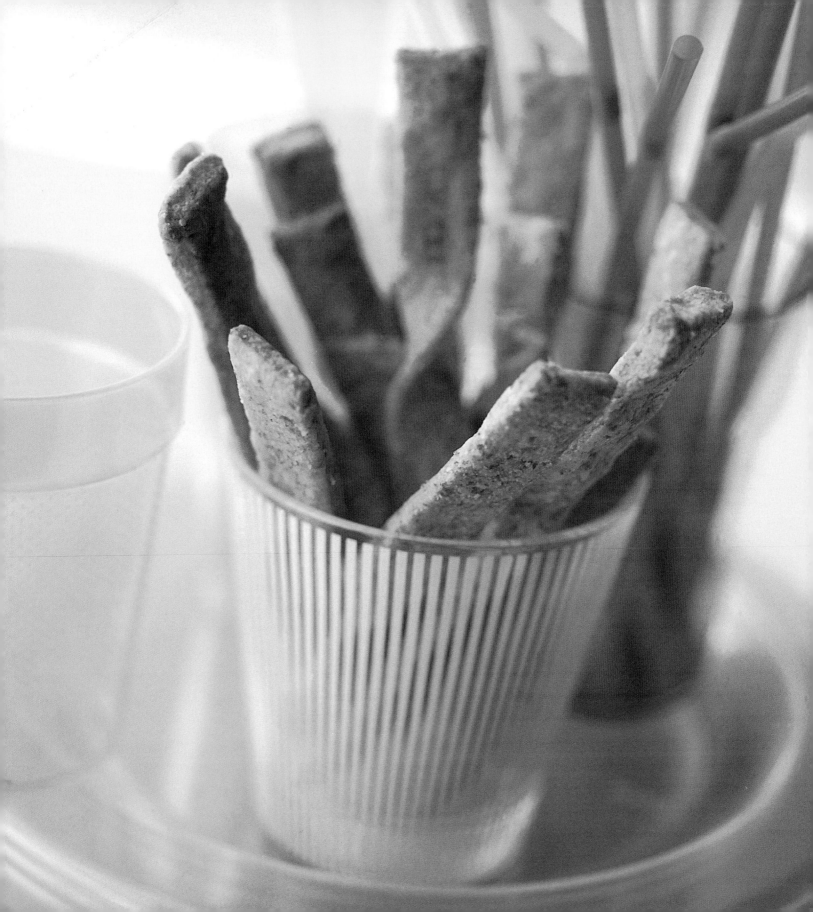

Time to Party

Many fun foods can help a children's party go with a swing. In addition to those in this chapter, you may like to offer some Dips, Dunkers & Nibbles (see page 116), Pizzas (see pages 52-4) and Wizard Drumsticks (see page 109), too. Sandwiches are often the last items children reach for, but you might have more success with original fillings (see page 112). Milk shakes are a good choice for drinks (see page 77), and you will almost certainly want to include some cakes and bakes (see pages 122-131).

CHEESE STRAWS

Cheese straws are one of life's small luxuries. Apart from being an excellent party food, they are also good for packed lunch boxes and picnics. Straws are quick and easy but, if you have time, shape the dough into hearts, rings, or even the first letter of each party guest's name. *Makes 30*

75 g (3 oz) wholemeal flour

50 g (2 oz) plain flour

100 g (3½ oz) butter, cut into small pieces

1 egg, separated

50 g (2 oz) Cheddar or Parmesan cheese, finely grated

pinch of cayenne pepper

½ teaspoon mustard powder (optional)

2 teaspoons poppy seeds (optional)

• Cheese straws keep well in an airtight tin for 3 or 4 days.
• If you make double the amount of cheese pastry, you can freeze half of it to roll out and cook for another occasion.

Combine the flours in a bowl and rub in the butter until the mixture resembles fine breadcrumbs. Add the egg yolk, cheese, cayenne, and mustard powder (if using). Stir with a fork, then knead lightly until smooth.

Roll out the cheese pastry on a floured work surface to a 5mm (¼ inch) thickness. Cut into long strips or 'straws' and brush with beaten egg white.

Give each strip a half-twist in the middle before laying on a lightly oiled baking tray. Sprinkle with poppy seeds (if using).

Bake in a preheated oven at 200°C (400°F) Gas Mark 6 for 10-12 minutes. Cool on a wire rack.

BONUS POINT
• Both flour and cheese contain calcium, which is essential for growing bones and teeth, and helps nerves and muscles function smoothly.

OKAY FOR UNDER-ONES?
4-6 months Not suitable. See pages 16-19 for other first food ideas.
6-12 months Use Cheddar rather than Parmesan. Crumble the cheese straw and soften with a little milk or water. Once your baby can cope, give them a cheese straw to hold, but supervise to make sure he or she doesn't poke themselves or anyone else in the eye!

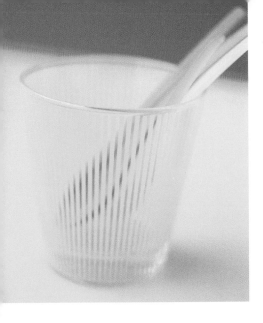

VEGETABLE CRISPS

Everyone seems to love the multicoloured vegetable crisps that you can buy nowadays in large – and expensive – bags. But it's easy to make them yourself, and cheaper too. In fact, it could hardly be a more effective way of encouraging children to eat vegetables! Choose a selection of colours – from deep pink beetroot, to orange sweet potato, to white celeriac – for optimum appeal. Brushing the vegetable slices with oil helps brings out their natural sweetness as they bake.

1 beetroot
½ sweet potato
2 carrots
1 parsnip
½ celeriac
corn or rapeseed (canola) oil for
  brushing

• For a treat, deep-fry rather than bake the vegetable slices, but go easy on your family's fat intake for the rest of that day. Deep-fried crisps look more like shop-bought ones than oven-baked crisps do.
• Heat 1 litre (1¾ pints) rapeseed (canola) oil in a deep-fryer or deep saucepan until a cube of bread dropped in immediately surfaces and sizzles. Deep-fry the vegetable slices in small batches until slightly browned; remove with a slotted spoon and drain (as above).
• WARNING If you are deep-frying, keep young children out of the room. Turn the pan-handle away from the front of the hob and never leave the oil unattended.

Peel the vegetables and cut into wafer-thin slices, no more than 1-2 mm (¹⁄₁₆ inch) thick. Pat the slices dry between double layers of kitchen paper, then place in a single layer on 2 baking trays.

Brush each vegetable slice lightly, but thoroughly, with a little oil. Turn the crisps over and brush the other sides with oil.

Bake in a preheated oven at 200°C (400°F) Gas Mark 6 for 10-12 minutes or until golden brown and cooked through. Celeriac, sweet potato and beetroot may need a further 1-2 minutes. (Note that beetroot colours only slightly; it shouldn't brown.) Transfer the crisps to a double layer of kitchen paper and leave to cool.

They will crisp up more on cooling, but should be served as soon as possible thereafter, otherwise they will start to soften. These crisps are ideal for dipping into Hummus (see page 138) and other Dips (see page 116).

BONUS POINTS
• Plant pigments in the vegetables act as antioxidants in the body, helping to protect cells from damage.
• The fibre in these crisps helps prevent constipation and also helps keep hormone levels healthy.

OKAY FOR UNDER-ONES?
4-9 months Not suitable. Give the plain vegetables boiled or steamed, and mashed with a little milk or water. Be warned that beetroot may colour your baby's urine and nappies slightly pink; this is quite normal.
9-12 months Once your baby can chew give crisps to hold, but stay close to hand in case a piece gets caught in the throat.

HERBY BREADSTICKS

Put a tumbler of breadsticks on the table and you'll soon find everyone tucking in. They are so easy that you may want to make them regularly, rather than just for parties. If you prefer plain breadsticks, just leave out the herbs. For a more distinctive herby flavour, double the quantity of herbs. Alternatively, for an original variation, try banana breadsticks (see tip box). *Makes 18-24*

150 g (5 oz) stoneground wholemeal bread flour

150 g (5 oz) strong white bread flour

1 sachet (7 g) easy-blend active dried yeast

4 tablespoons olive oil, plus a little extra for brushing

2 teaspoons dried mixed herbs

100 ml (3½ fl oz) warm water

Put the flours into a large bowl and stir in the yeast. Make a well in the middle and add the oil, herbs, and most of the water. Stir well, then knead for 5-10 minutes, adding the rest of the water if needed to form a smooth, pliable dough. Place in a clean bowl, cover with a damp cloth and leave in a warm place for about 1 hour, or until doubled in size.

Knead the dough again, then divide it into 24 small pieces. Roll each one into a long thin stick. Place the sticks, well apart, on 2 oiled baking trays and brush them with oil. Leave for 10 minutes in a warm place, then bake in a preheated oven at 180°C (350°F) Gas Mark 4 for 12-15 minutes, or until golden brown.

Serve these breadsticks on their own, or with Dips (see page 116). You can also pop some into a packed lunch box with a tub of dip.

BONUS POINTS
• Both flour and yeast are good sources of vitamin B, needed for healthy nerves.
• Wholemeal flour contains fibre which helps keep the bowel healthy.

OKAY FOR UNDER-ONES?
4-6 months Not suitable. See pages 16-19 for other first food ideas.
6-12 months Crumble a breadstick and soften with a little milk or water. Or, once your baby can manage, offer them a breadstick to hold and suck or bite, but supervise carefully to make sure he or she doesn't poke themselves or anyone else in the eye!

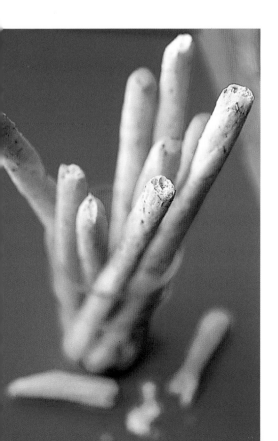

> • For banana breadsticks, replace the herbs with 1 banana, well mashed. Add a little less water to begin with, as you'll need to use less overall.

HUMMUS

425 g (14 oz) canned chickpeas, drained
3 tablespoons tahini (see tip box)
1 garlic clove, crushed
1 tablespoon sesame oil
juice of ½ lemon
a little water to mix (if required)

Hummus is excellent for dipping into at parties, and it's also a popular packed lunch item to provide in a little plastic tub. Originally a Middle-eastern favourite, this tasty dip is now universally popular. The main ingredient is chickpeas, which are puréed with sesame seeds or sesame seed paste, garlic and lemon juice. Flavourings can be adjusted to suit individual tastes.

Put the chickpeas in an electric blender or a food processor with the tahini, garlic, sesame oil and lemon juice. Blend until smooth, adding a little water if necessary so the texture is easily spoonable.

Serve with Herby breadsticks (see page 137), pitta bread, raw carrot or celery sticks.

BONUS POINTS
• Chickpeas are rich in protein, fibre, calcium and iron.
• Sesame seeds offer protein, calcium, iron, and the essential omega-6 fatty acid – linoleic acid – that is especially good for skin, hair and nails.

OKAY FOR UNDER-ONES?
4-6 months Not suitable. Instead, give some cooked carrot mashed with a little milk or water.
6-12 months Use freshly cooked chickpeas (see tip box), rather than canned ones which have added salt.

> • Tahini – ready-made sesame-seed paste – is available from larger supermarkets and healthfood stores. If unobtainable, replace with 2 tablespoons of sesame seeds and use an extra 1 tablespoon of sesame oil.
>
> • Dried chickpeas can be used in place of canned ones, and have the advantage that they do not contain added salt. However, you will need to soak them overnight in cold water before cooking. The next day, drain the chickpeas and place in a large saucepan. Add fresh cold water to cover, bring to the boil and fast boil for 10 minutes, then lower the heat and simmer for 1½-2 hours until tender. Drain thoroughly and use as above.

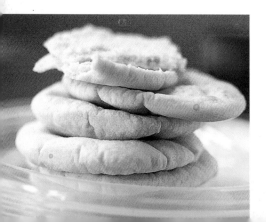

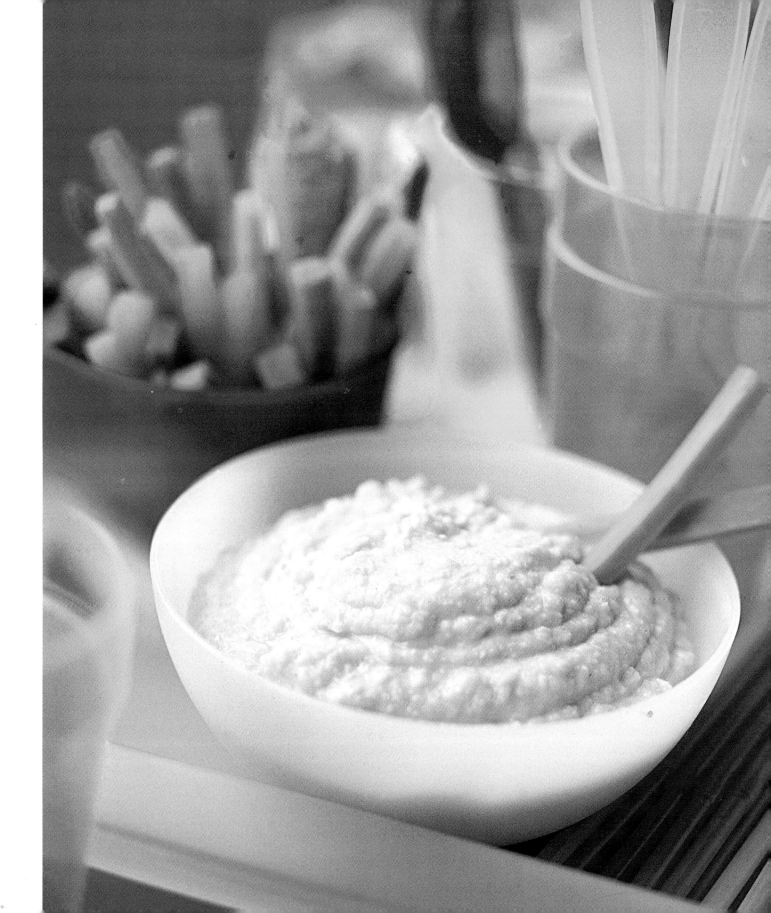

PUFFED TOMATO TARTLETS

Red and gold colours stimulate the appetite, so expect these little tomato tarts to be popular. Buy ready-made chilled or frozen puff pastry for ease and speed, but remember to allow 2 hours for frozen pastry to defrost before rolling out. *Makes about 15*

250 g (8 oz) ready-made puff pastry
(fresh or frozen and thawed)
1 egg, beaten
250 g (8 oz) cherry tomatoes, sliced
4 teaspoons olive oil
4 teaspoons Parmesan or Cheddar
cheese

Roll out the pastry on a lightly floured surface to a large rectangle, 3-5 mm (⅛-¼ inch) in thickness. Using a 5 cm (2 inch) pastry cutter, cut out about 15 pastry rounds.

Place the pastry rounds on a baking sheet and prick with a fork, leaving a small margin at the edge. Brush the rounds with beaten egg. Lay the tomato slices on top, leaving the margins free.

Brush the tomatoes with olive oil and sprinkle with Parmesan or Cheddar. Bake in a preheated oven at 200°C (400°F) Gas Mark 6 for 15 minutes, or until the pastry rims are puffed and golden brown.

BONUS POINTS
Tomatoes are rich in the plant pigment – lycopene. This acts as an antioxidant in the body, helping to protect cells from damage. Tomato lycopene is most readily available to us when tomatoes are cooked, as here, with a little fat.

OKAY FOR UNDER-ONES?
4-6 months Not suitable. See pages 16-19 for other first food ideas.
6-12 months Use homemade pastry, rather than ready-made which contains salt – it doesn't have to be puff. Don't use Parmesan, as it is a relatively salty cheese. Blend the food with a little milk or water. Once your baby can chew, cut the tartlet up small.

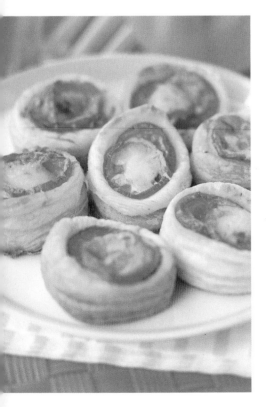

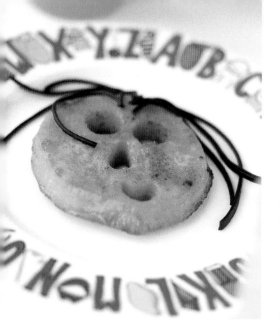

PUMPKIN FACES

These are fun to make for children when pumpkins are in season. You simply cut rounds of pumpkin and make holes for eyes, nose and mouth. Once baked and given shiny black bootlace 'hair', they look terrific.

1 pumpkin, halved, peeled and
    deseeded
50 g (2 oz) demerara sugar
50 g (2 oz) butter, cut into little pieces
4 tablespoons orange juice
pinch of powdered cinnamon or cloves
4 liquorice 'bootlaces'

Using a sharp knife, cut rounds from the pumpkin for 'faces'. Carefully make holes for the eyes, nose and mouth, using the knife and an apple corer.

Lay the 'faces' in greased shallow roasting tins and sprinkle with the sugar, butter, orange juice and cinnamon. Bake in a preheated oven at 180°C (350°F) Gas Mark 4 for 30 minutes, basting halfway through cooking.

Carefully transfer each pumpkin 'face' to a plate and allow to cool. Arrange a few pieces of liquorice bootlace around the top to resemble 'hair'.

BONUS POINT
Pumpkin is rich in beta-carotene, an orange-yellow antioxidant plant pigment that helps protect every body cell from damage, but is particularly protective to the eyes, and the linings of the mouth, throat, digestive tract and urinary tract.

OKAY FOR UNDER-ONES?
4-6 months Not suitable. Instead, blend some plain baked pumpkin with a little milk or fruit juice.
6-12 months Not suitable. Mash baked pumpkin, or cut it into pieces.

BACON-WRAPPED PRUNES

6 rashers streaky bacon, derinded
12 'ready-to-eat' stoned prunes

Bacon-wrapped prunes are great party food. Simply, wrap halved bacon rashers around prunes, place on an oiled baking tray and cook in a preheated oven at 180°C (350°F) Gas Mark 4 for about 20 minutes.

BONUS POINT
• Prunes have a high ability to mop up 'free radicals' – unstable oxygen particles formed in the body by such things as a poor diet and too much sun, which can promote heart disease, strokes, premature ageing and cancer.

OKAY FOR UNDER-ONES?
Not suitable.

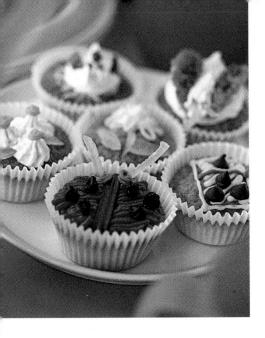

FAIRY CAKES

Pretty little iced fairy cakes are always popular at parties, especially when they are attractively decorated. Create a variety of different patterns, or spread icing smoothly on the cakes and write each guest's name on top with easy-to-use tubes of writing icing (available from the home baking section of most supermarkets). As a variation, add 50 g (2 oz) of chopped dried cherries or apricots, or sultanas, to the cake mixture. To make butterfly cakes, cut a slice off the top of each cake, halve and attach to the cake at an angle with icing to resemble wings. *Makes 16-18*

1½ tablespoons milk

3 eggs

150 g (5 oz) caster sugar

125 g (4 oz) self-raising flour

75 g (3 oz) butter, melted

Cream cheese frosting:

75 g (3 oz) low-fat cream cheese

50 g (2 oz) icing sugar

Glacé icing:

150 g (5 oz) icing sugar

2-3 teaspoons water

2-3 teaspoons lemon juice

To decorate:

tubes of coloured writing icing

chopped dried papaya or apricot

chocolate buttons or chocolate drops

angelica or crystallized ginger (optional)

Whisk the milk, eggs and sugar together in a bowl for 4-5 minutes, until pale and thick. Carefully fold in the flour, followed by the butter. Line 16-18 sections of two 12-hole bun tins with paper cases. Spoon the mixture into the cases, so they are just over half full. Bake in a preheated oven at 180°C (350°F) Gas Mark 4 for 10-15 minutes, or until risen and golden brown. Transfer to a wire rack to cool.

To make cream cheese frosting, mix the cream cheese and icing sugar together until smooth.

To make glacé icing, mix the icing sugar with sufficient water and lemon juice to make a smooth icing that has a piping consistency. Pipe or spoon the icing(s) on top of the cakes and apply the decorations to create a variety of patterns. Or smooth icing on top of the cakes and pipe on the children's names. Leave to set for several hours, if possible.

OKAY FOR UNDER-ONES?
4-6 months Not suitable. See pages 16-19 for other first food ideas.
6-9 months Best avoided, as a baby of this age won't know what he or she is missing.
9-12 months Ideally, under-ones shouldn't have added sugar. However, a very occasional fairy cake – preferably without icing, and certainly without applied decorations – won't hurt. Give your baby the cake if he or she is old enough to hold it, and clean teeth and gums afterwards.

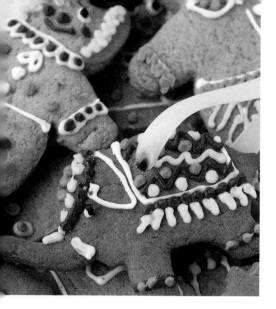

GINGERBREAD BISCUITS

Gingerbread biscuits are easy to make and keep well. At Christmas time, decorate with icing, thread with festive ribbon and hang them on the Christmas tree (see tip box). For a birthday party, ice each child's name on a biscuit. Either arrange on a tray or pop into party bags for children to take home. *Makes 12-16*

75 g (3 oz) golden syrup

65 g (2½ oz) granulated sugar

1 teaspoon ground ginger

½ teaspoon ground cinnamon

¼ teaspoon ground cloves (optional)

65 g (2½ oz) butter

1 teaspoon bicarbonate of soda

2 teaspoons water

1 egg, beaten

300 g (10 oz) plain flour

Icing (optional):

100 g (3½ oz) icing sugar

1 egg white, lightly beaten

few drops of food colouring (optional)

• For festive biscuits to hang on the tree, cut out Christmas trees or stars, using suitable cutters. Before baking, make a hole in the top of each one with a chopstick or skewer, at least 1 cm (½ inch) from the edge, making sure the hole is big enough to take the ribbon. After baking and cooling, thread a 25 cm (10 inch) length of ribbon through each biscuit and knot the ends.

Put the golden syrup, sugar and spices in a heavy-based pan and heat gently, stirring, until the sugar melts. Add the butter and stir until melted. Leave to cool for 10 minutes.

Dissolved the bicarbonate of soda in 2 teaspoons water. Add to the syrup mixture with the egg and flour. Stir well and mix to a smooth dough, then wrap in clingfilm and leave to rest in a cool place for 1 hour.

Roll out the dough on a lightly floured surface to a 3 mm (⅛ inch) thickness. Cut out rounds or other shapes, using biscuit cutters or a knife, and place on lightly greased baking sheets.

Bake in a preheated oven at 220°C (425°F) Gas Mark 7 for 10-15 minutes until golden brown. Leave on the baking sheets for 1 minute, then loosen the biscuits with a palette knife and transfer to a wire rack to cool.

To make the icing (if required), put the icing sugar in a bowl and stir in the egg white, a little at a time, to make a smooth thick icing that has a piping consistency. Mix in a few drops of colouring (if using). Spoon into a piping bag and pipe on to the biscuits decoratively.

Serve gingerbread biscuits on their own, or as an accompaniment to apple purée or stewed rhubarb or plums.

OKAY FOR UNDER-ONES?

4-6 months Not suitable. Instead, give stewed eating apple, or mashed raw dessert pear, mixed with a little milk or water.

6-9 months Best avoided completely, as a baby of this age won't know what he or she is missing.

9-12 months Ideally, under-ones shouldn't have added sugar. However, the occasional gingerbread biscuit – perhaps once a week – won't hurt, provided you clean the teeth and gums afterwards. Wait until your baby is old enough to hold a biscuit and expect them to take a little time to get used to the spiciness. Alternatively, offer them some homemade rusks (see page 19).

Index